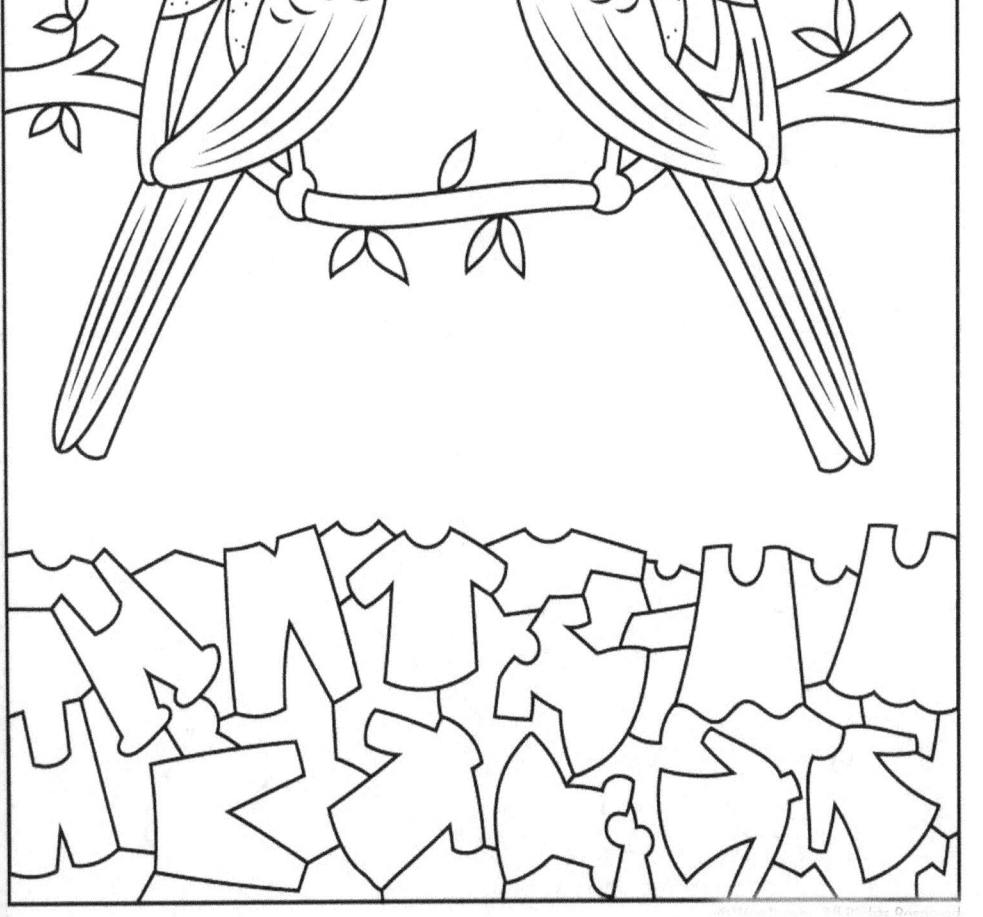

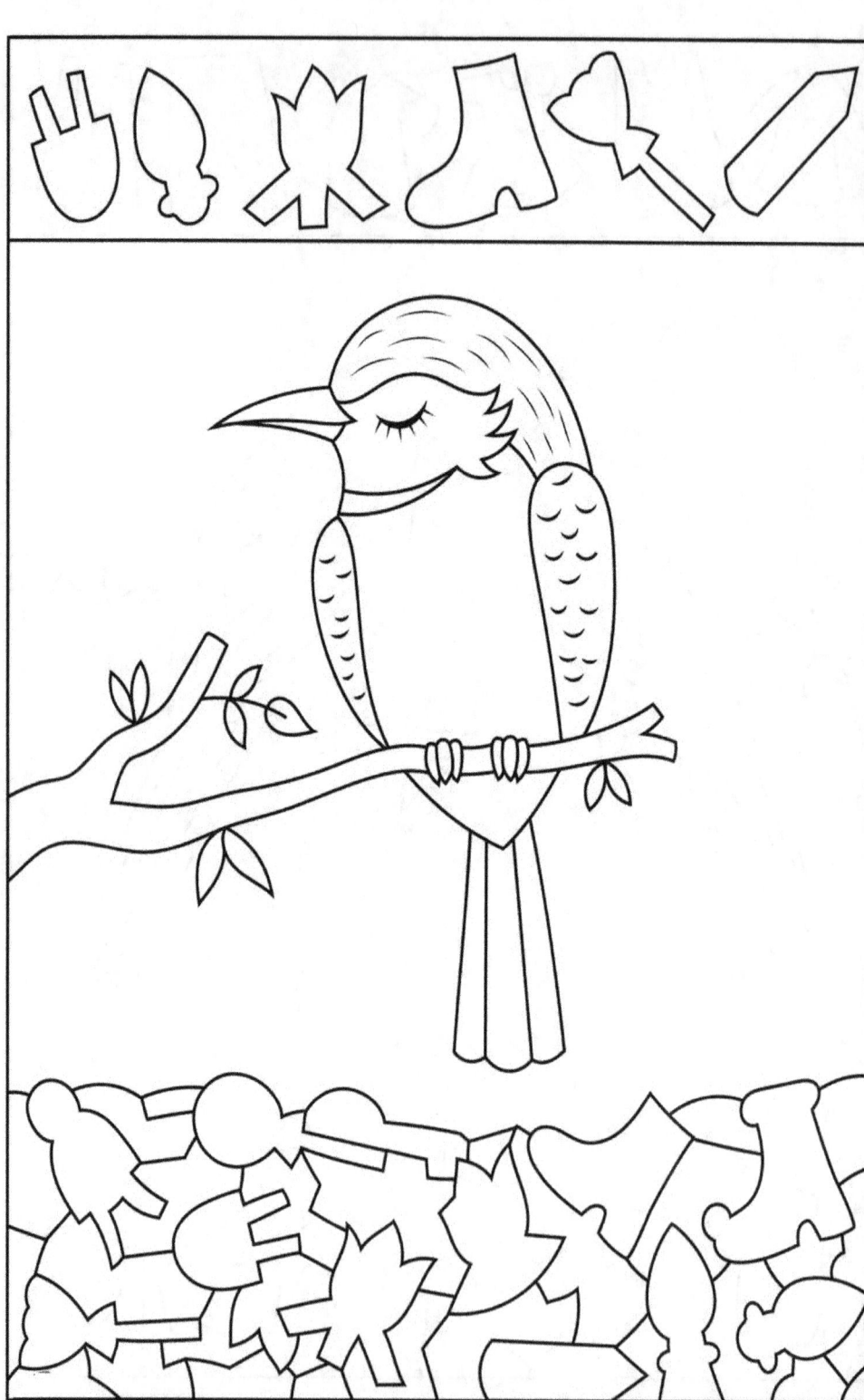

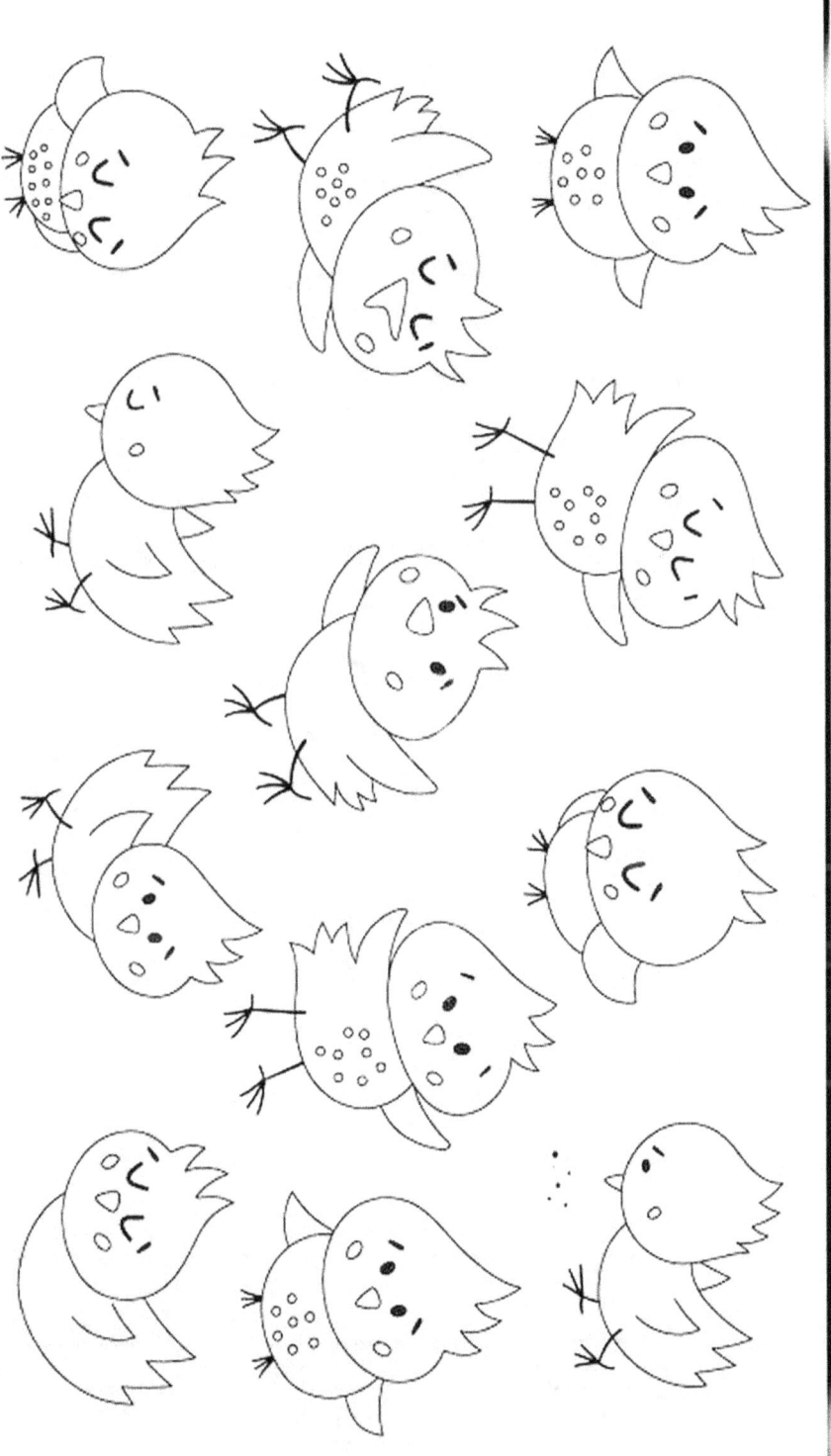

FIND TWO SAME CHICKS

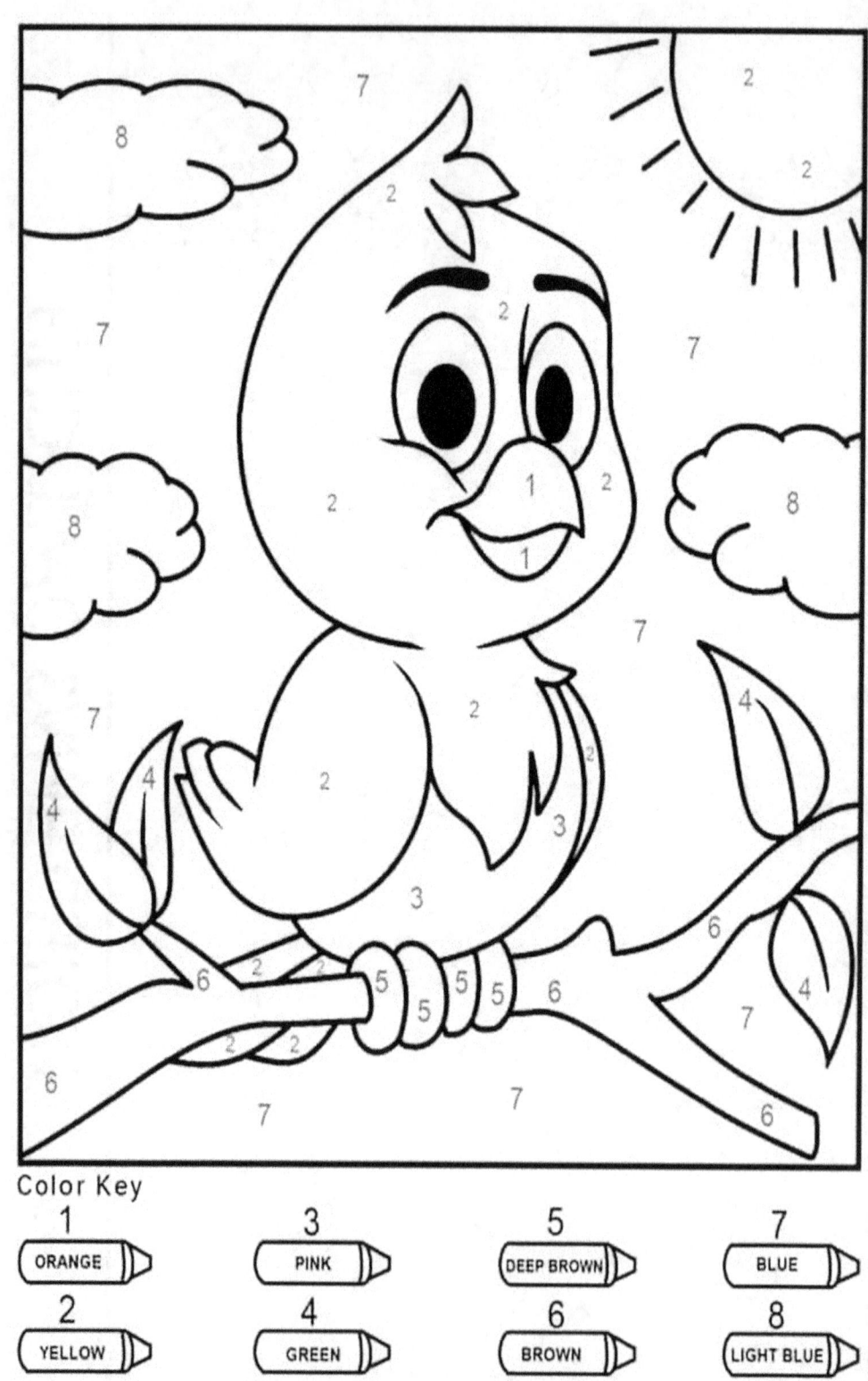

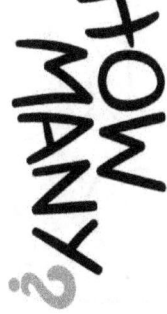

HOW MANY?

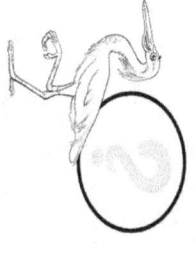
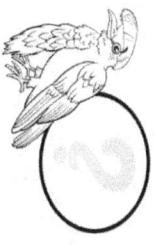

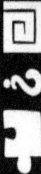

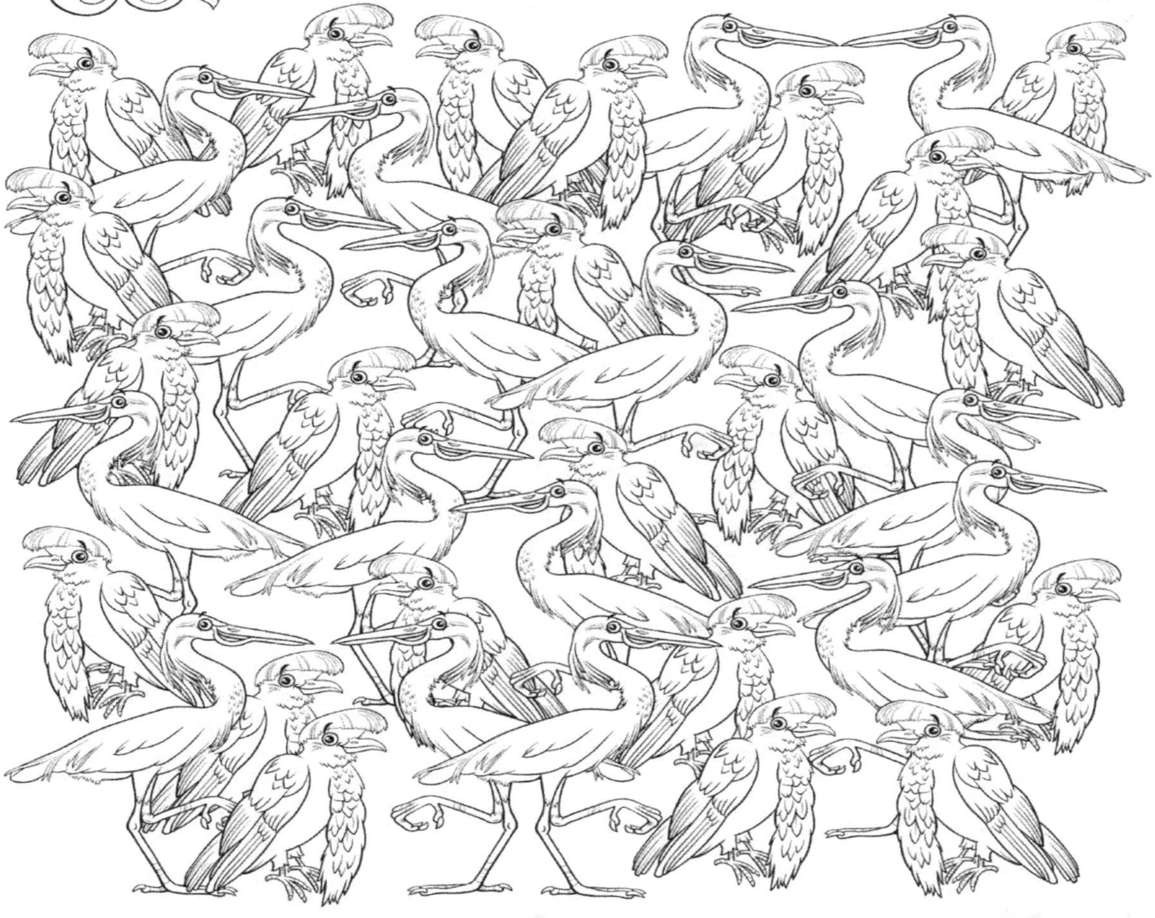

ANSWER

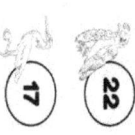

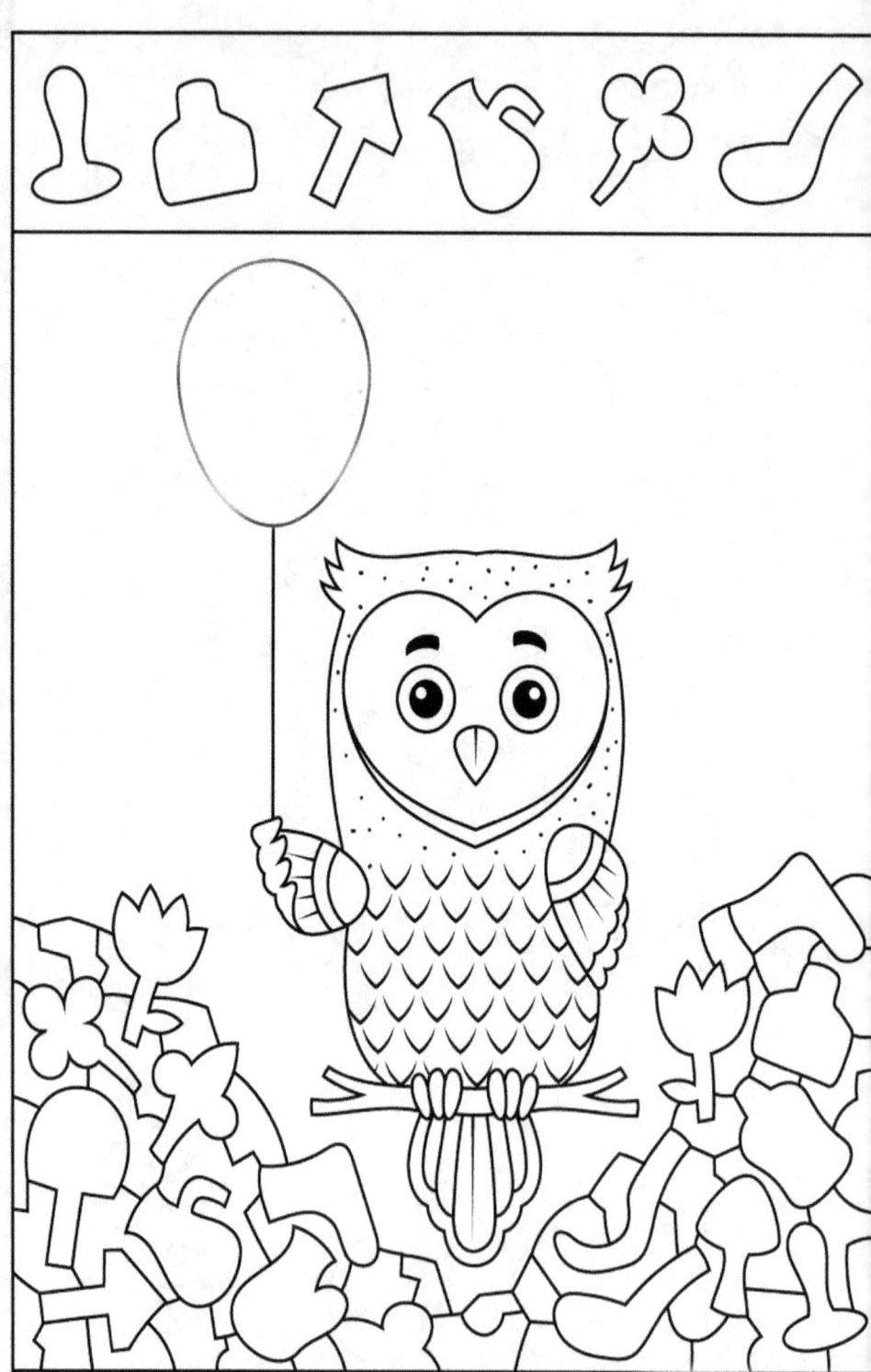

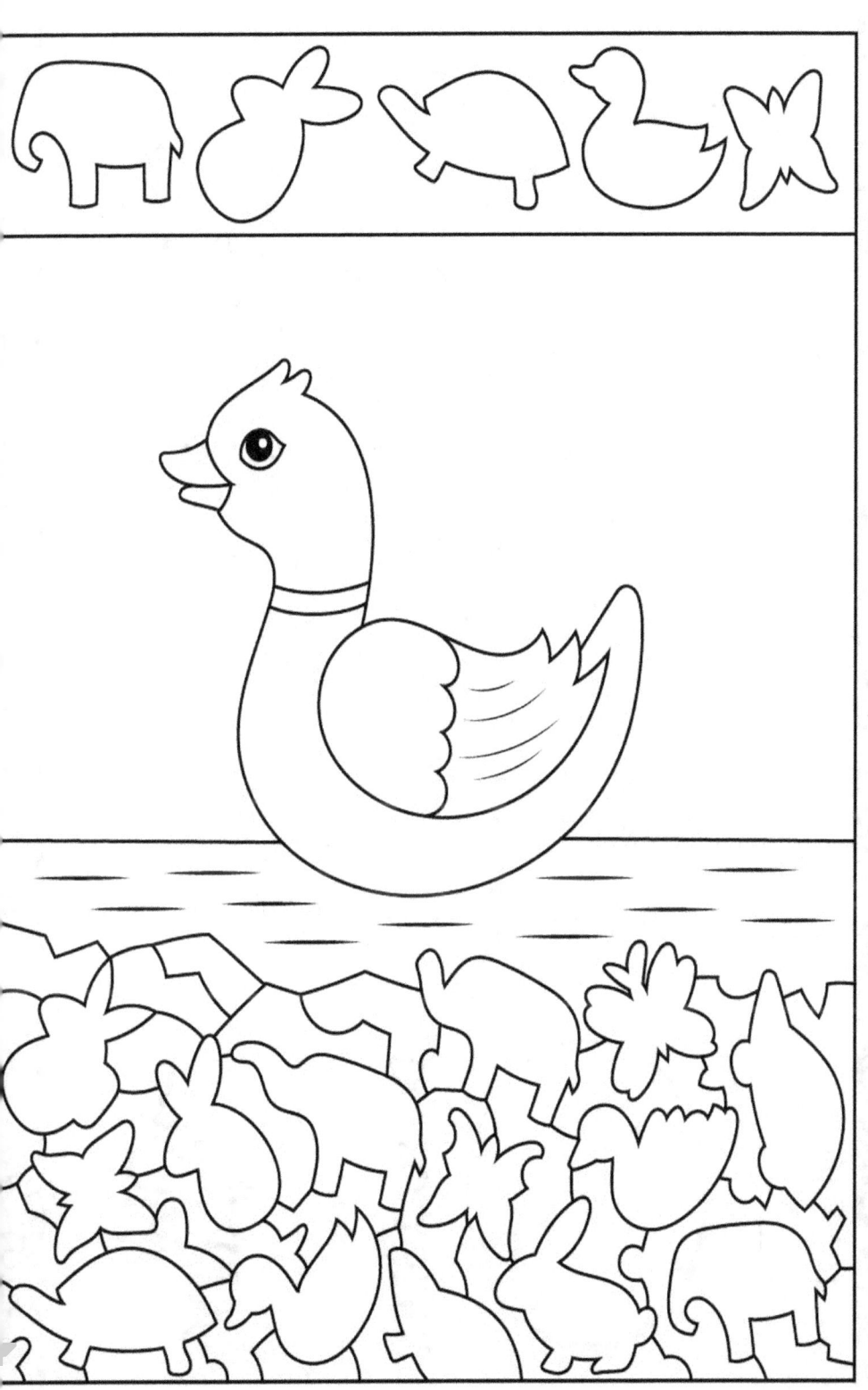

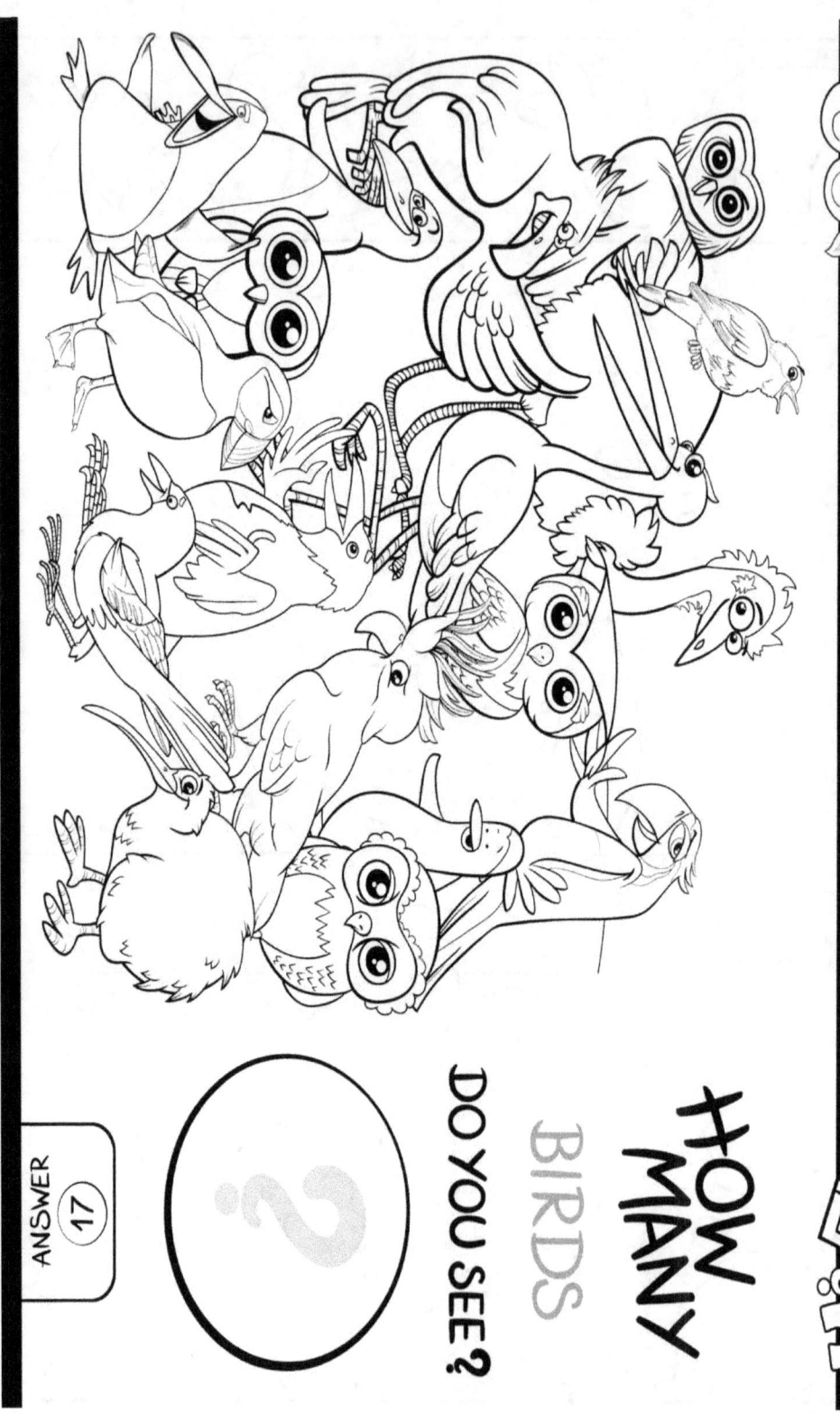

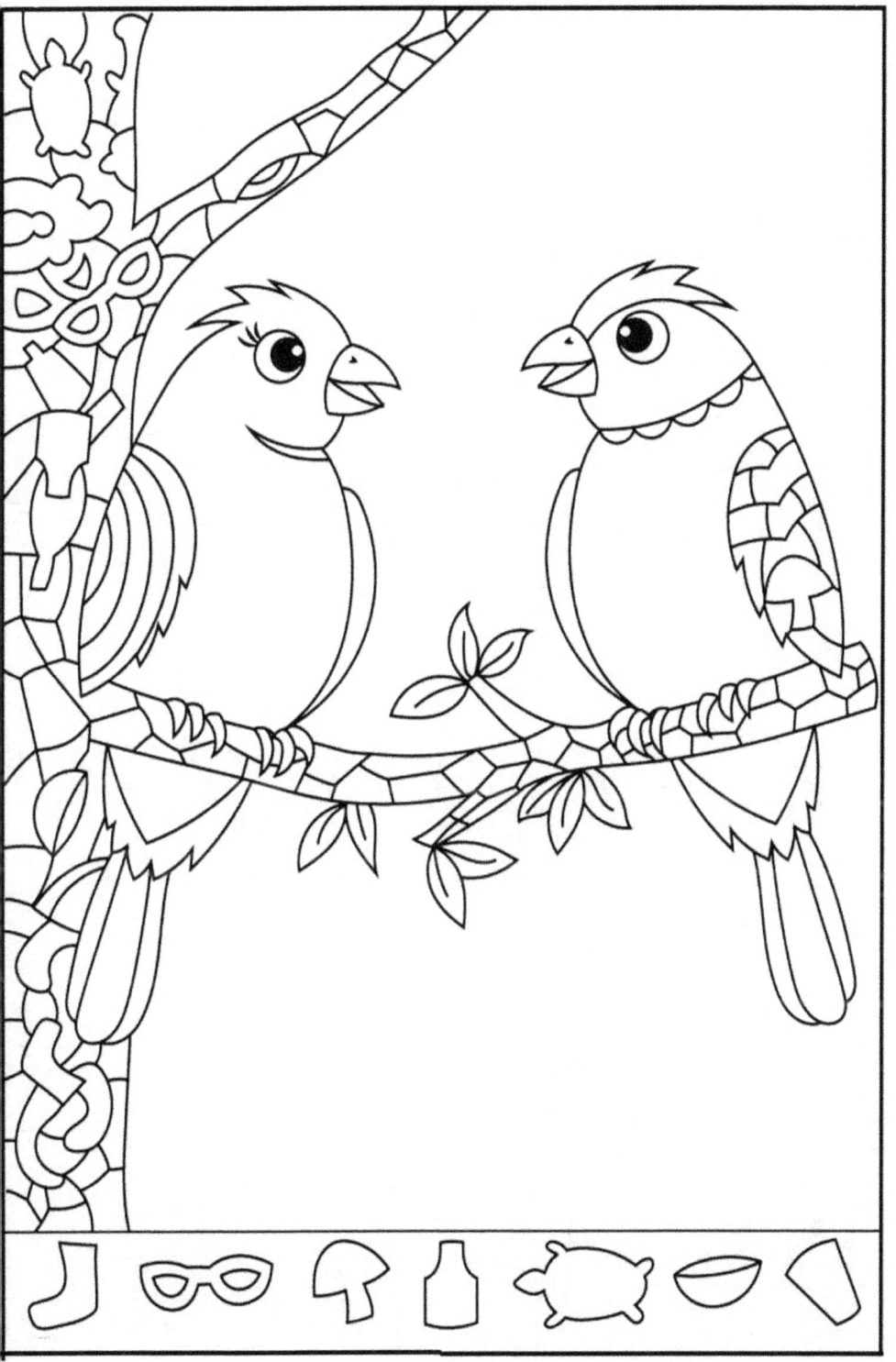

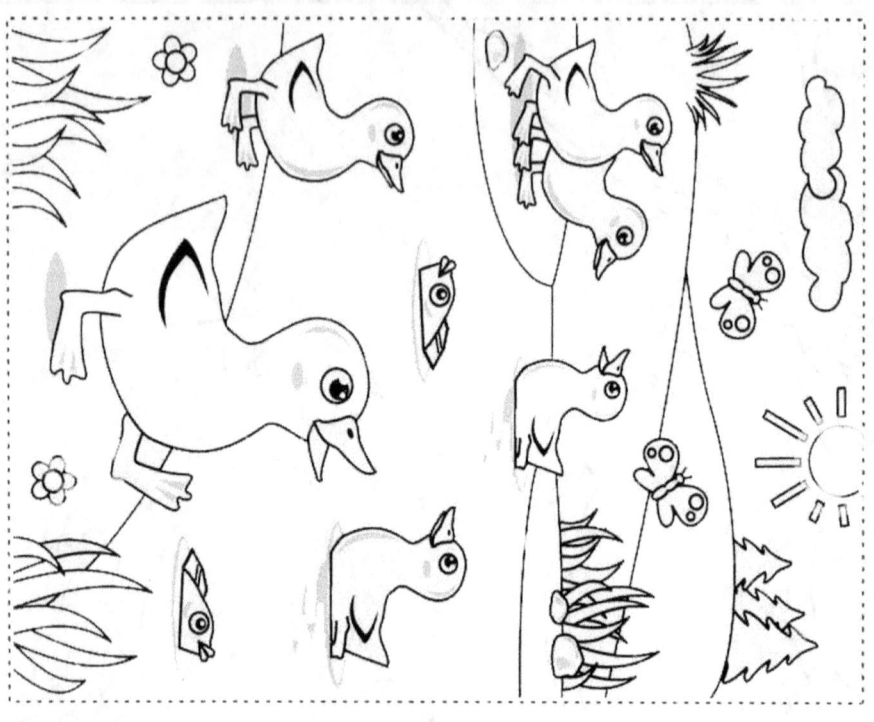
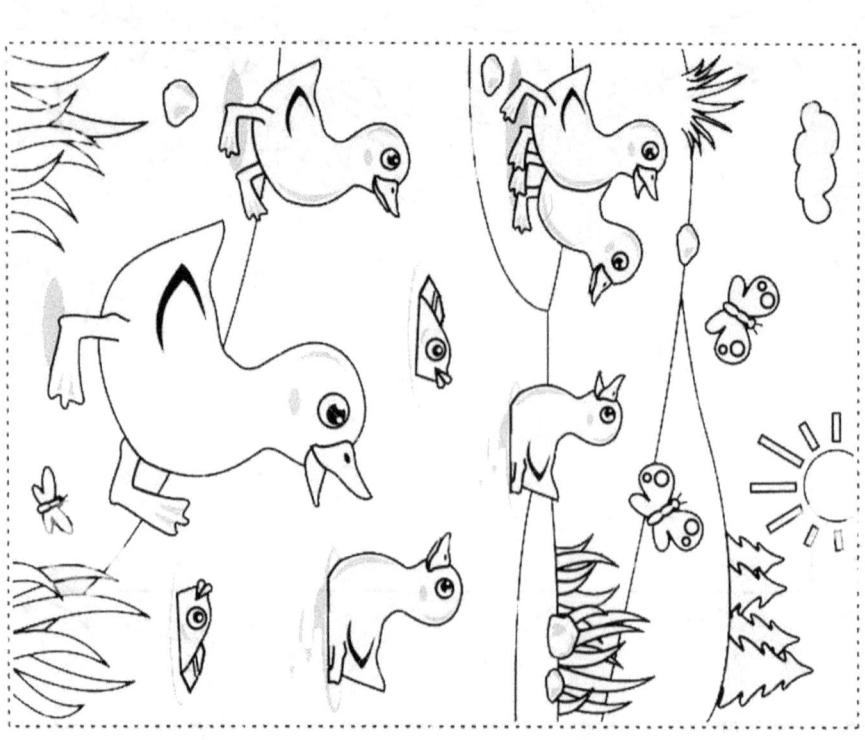

Find the ten differences between the two pictures.

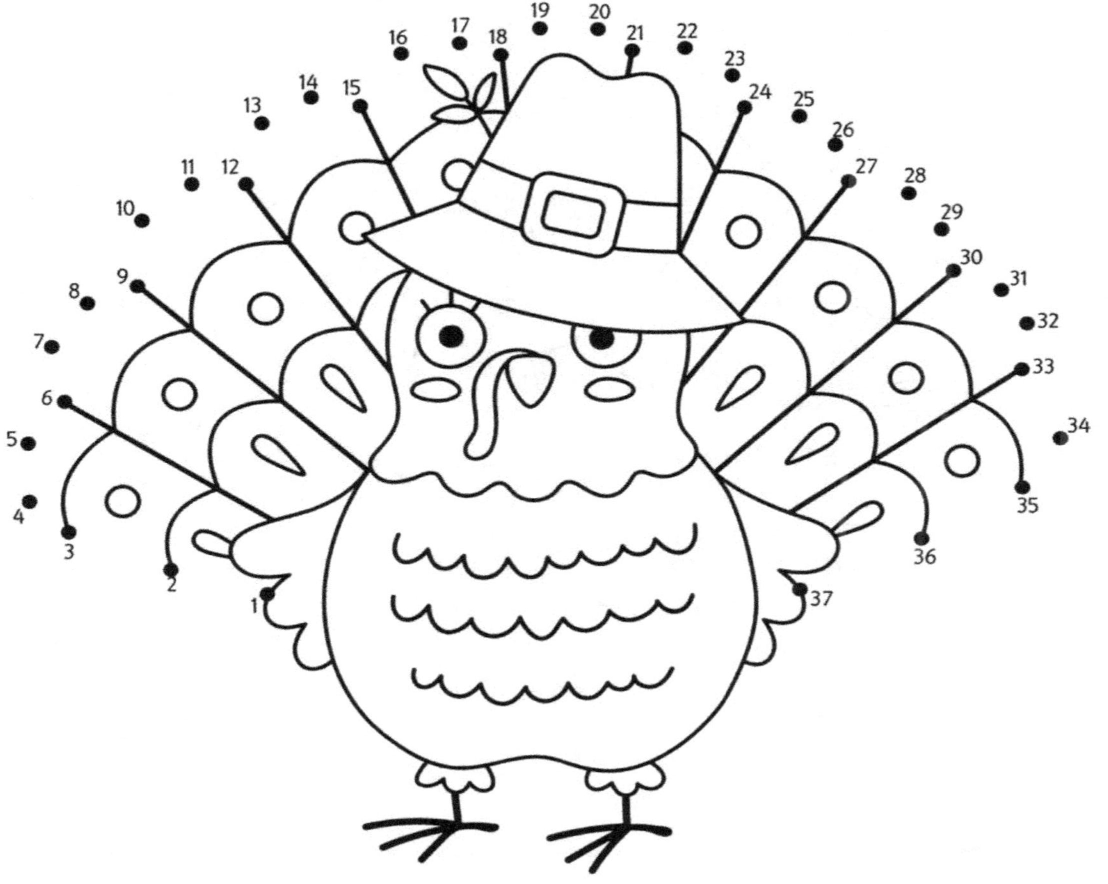

Connect the Dots

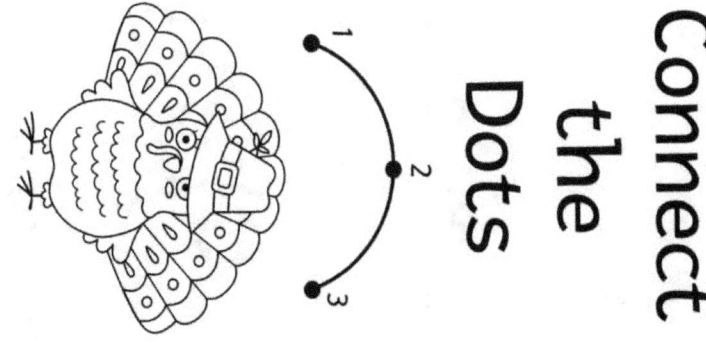

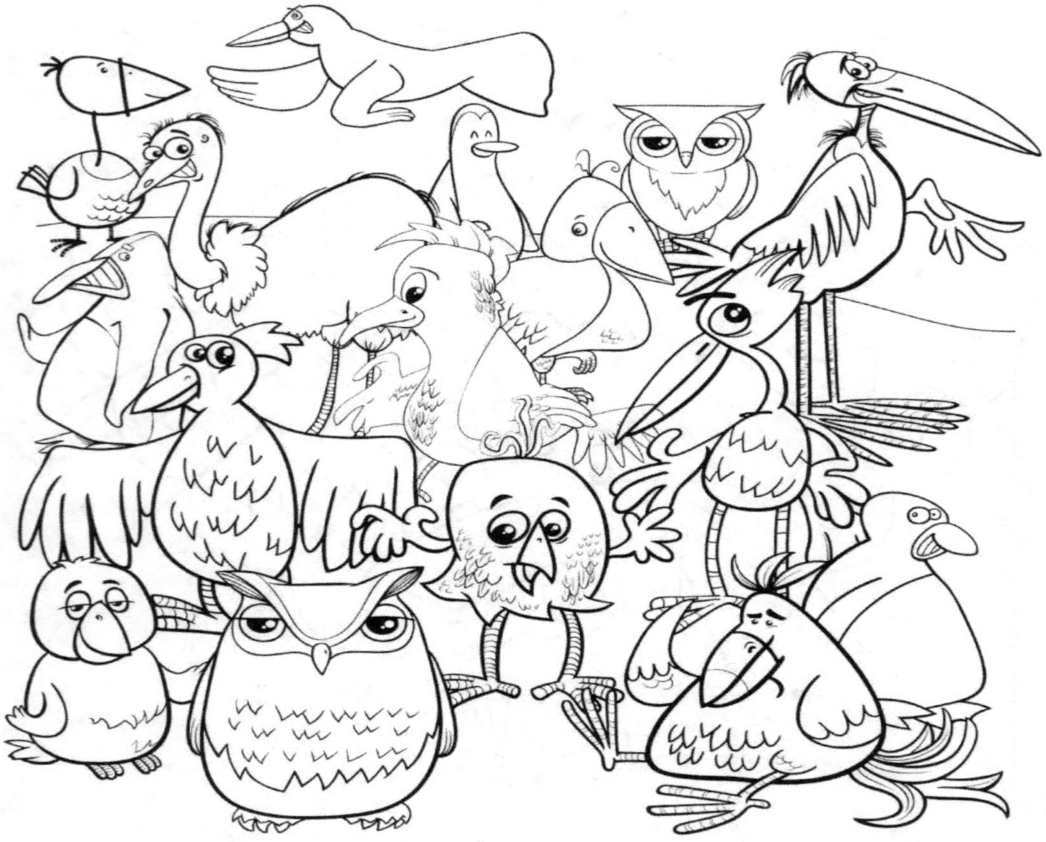

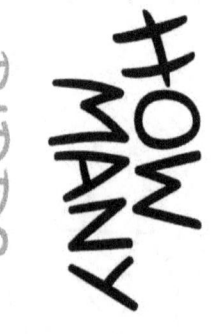

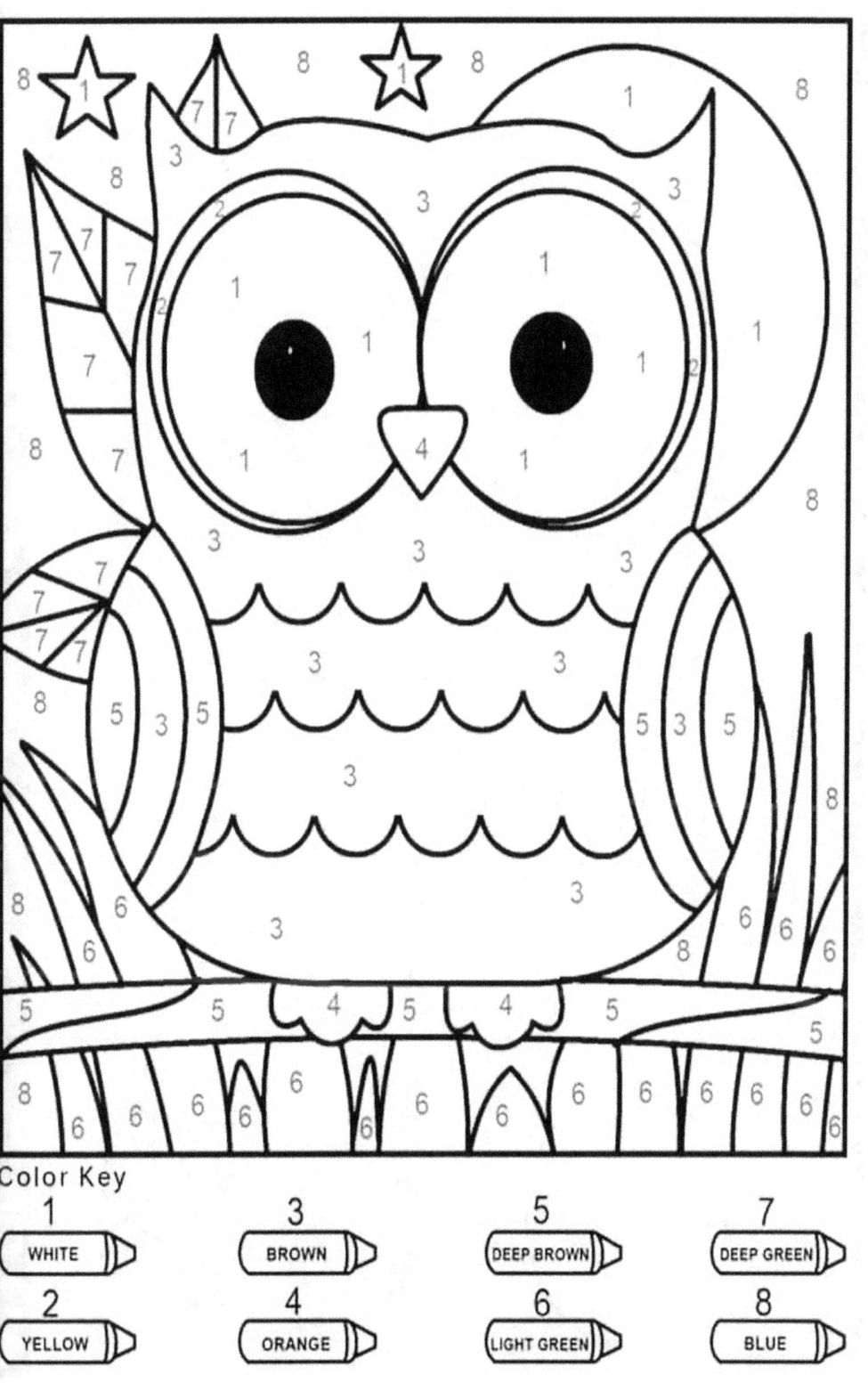

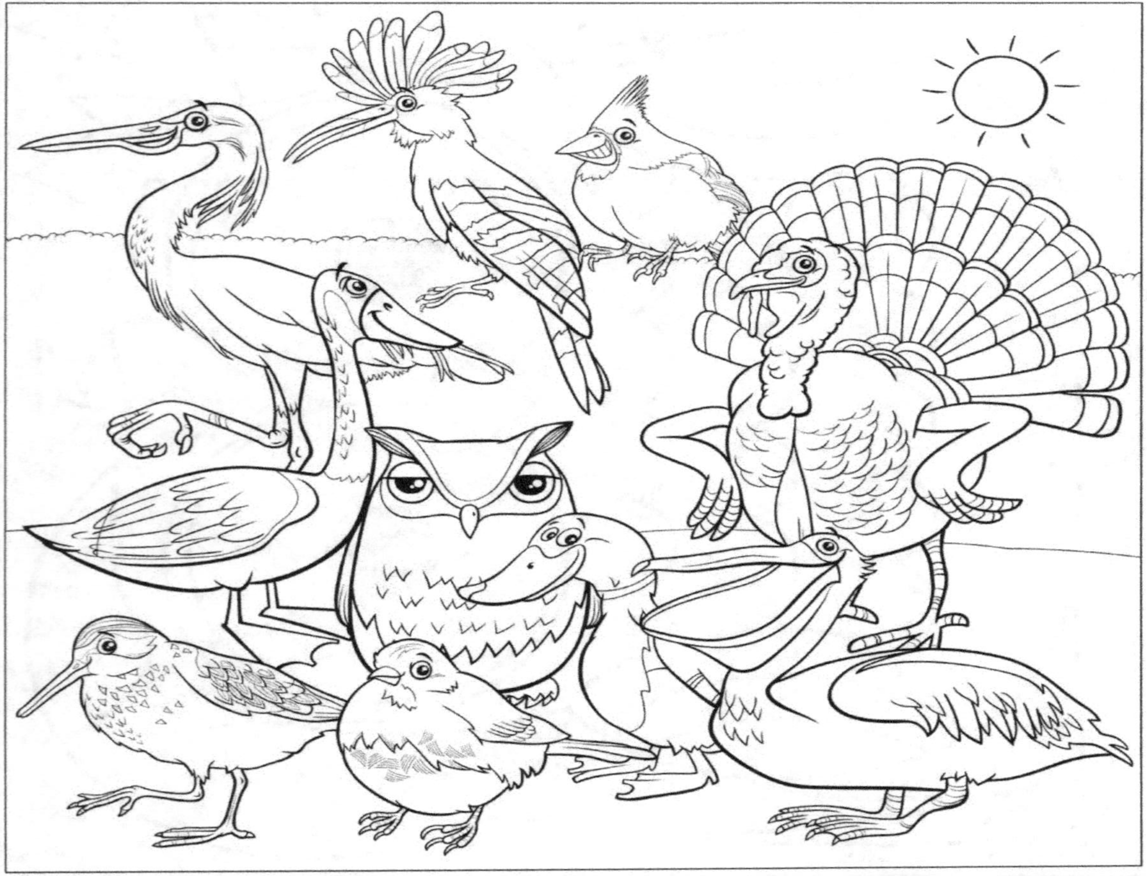

HOW MANY BIRDS DO YOU SEE?

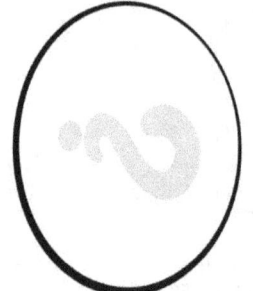

ANSWER 10

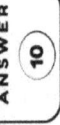

ACTIVITY SHEET

Handwriting practise - Good morning!

Contour sun rays and fence. Color the picture.

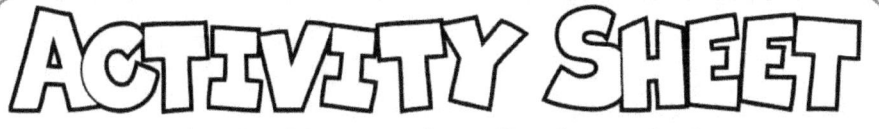

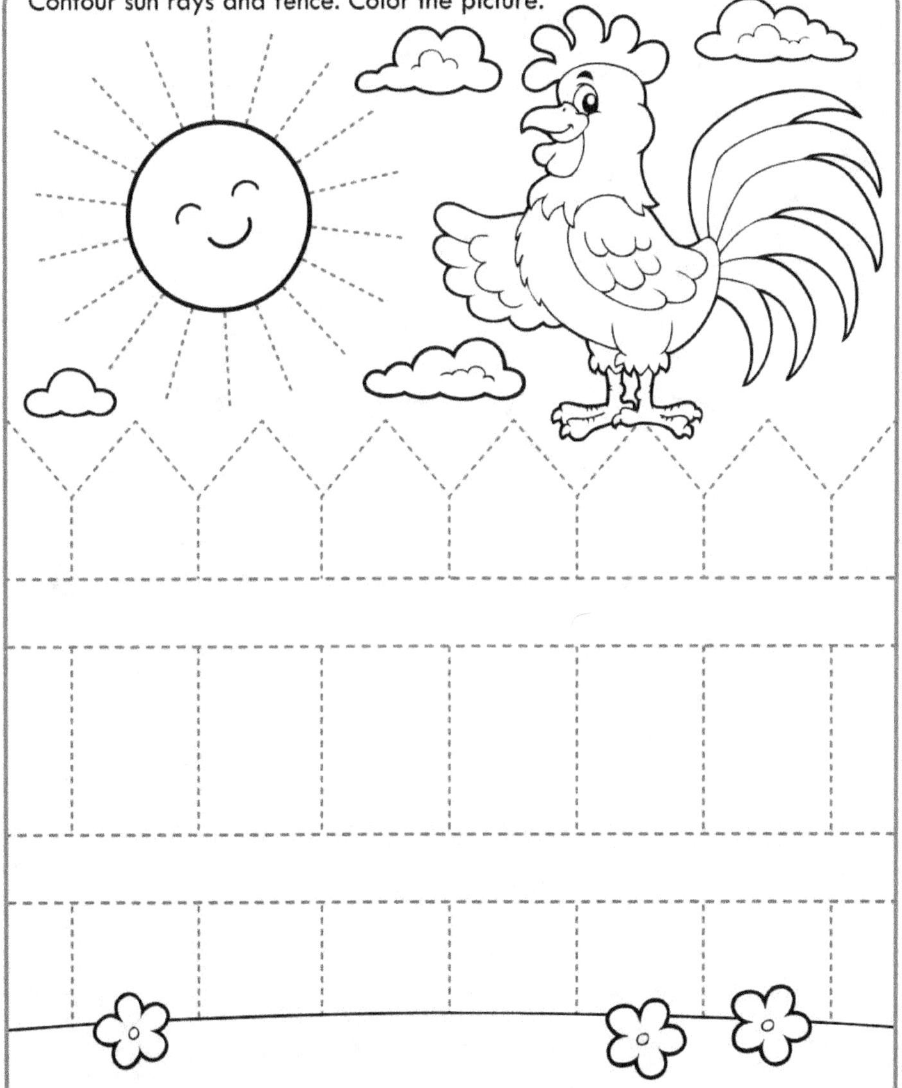

Shapes Maze!

Color in the ⬭'s to find the path to the pond.

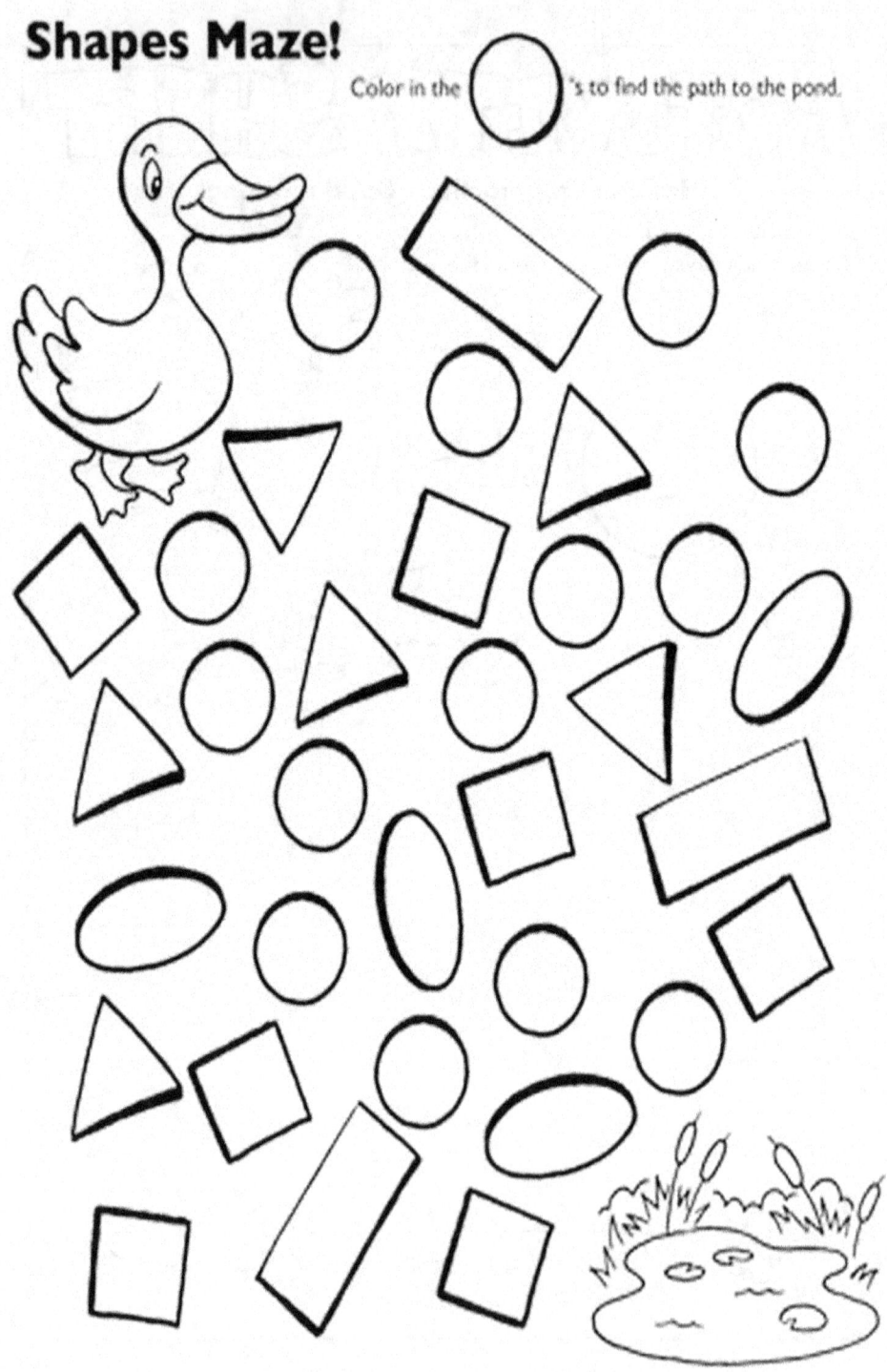

HOW MANY?

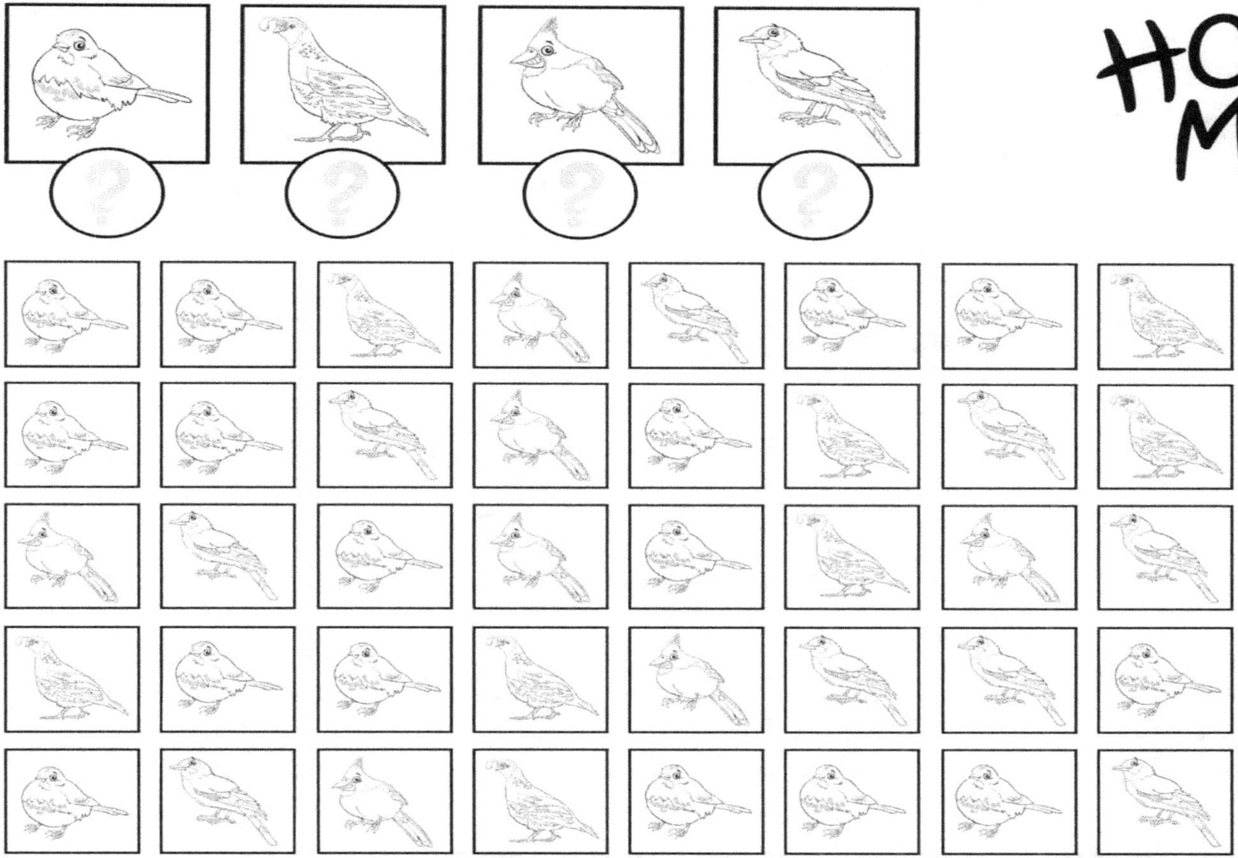

ANSWER
16 | 8 | 7 | 9

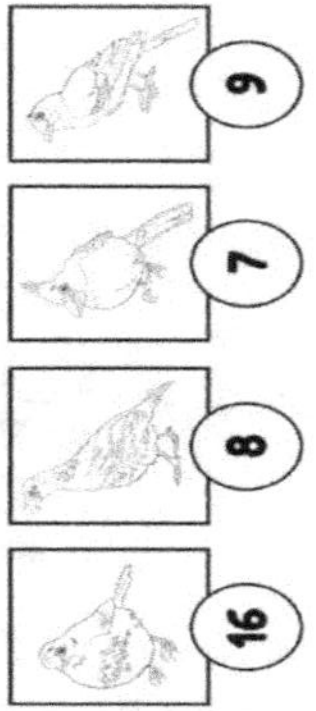

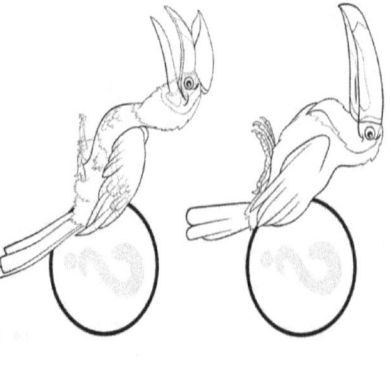

HOW MANY?

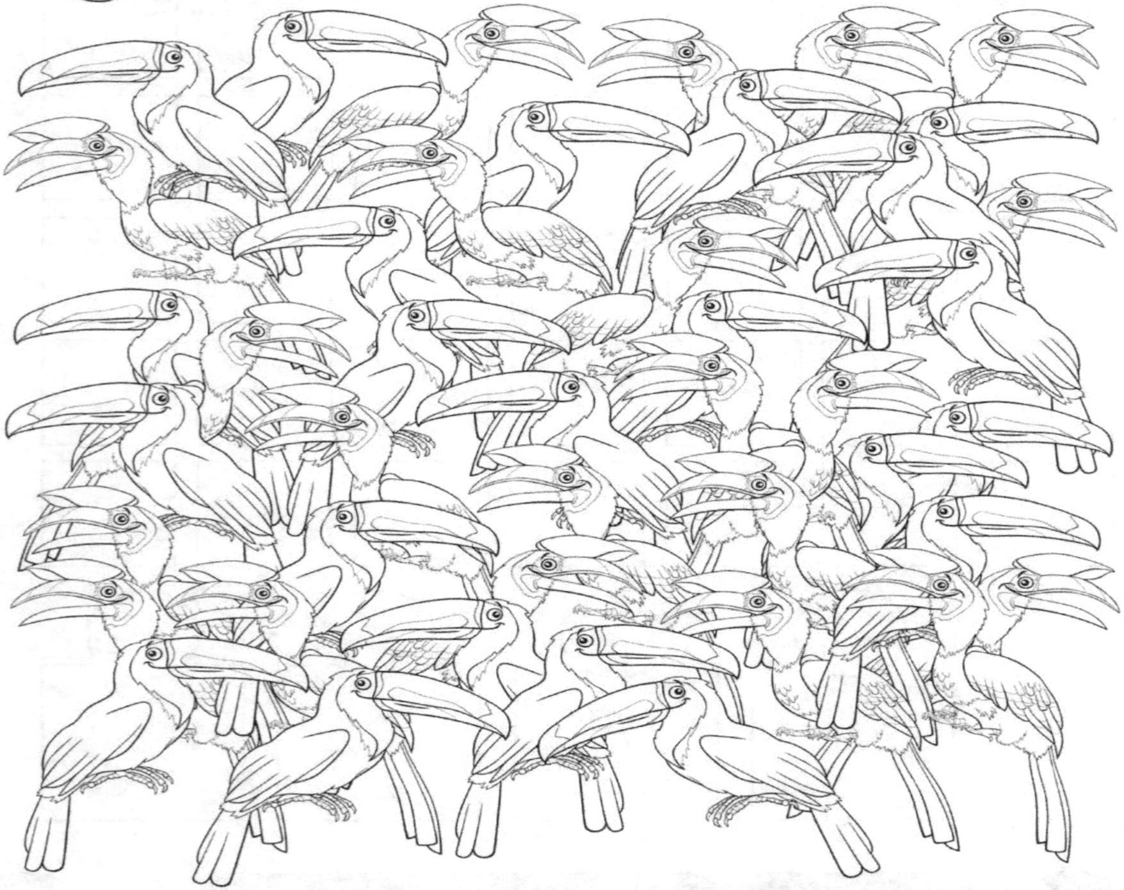

ANSWER
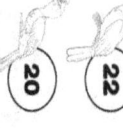
20 22

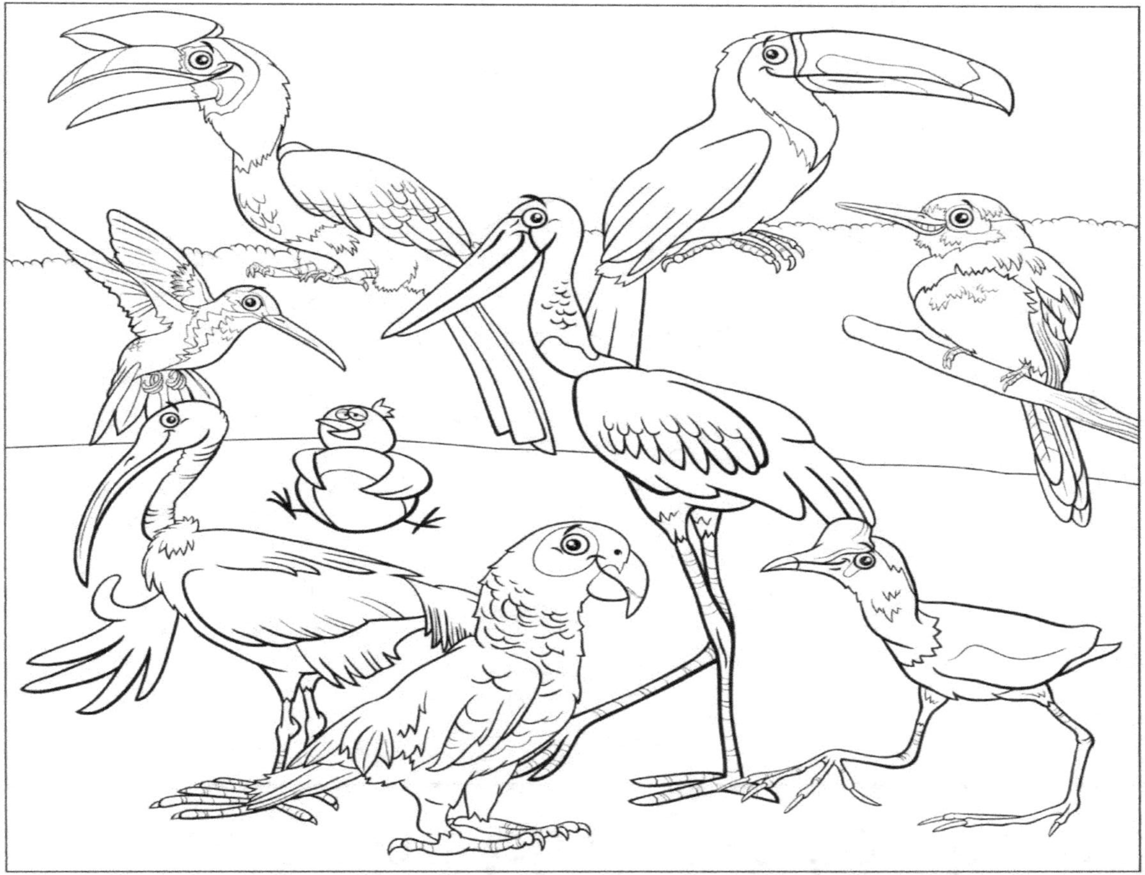

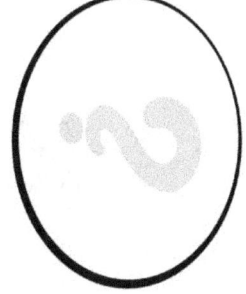

HOW MANY?
BIRDS DO YOU SEE?

ANSWER
9

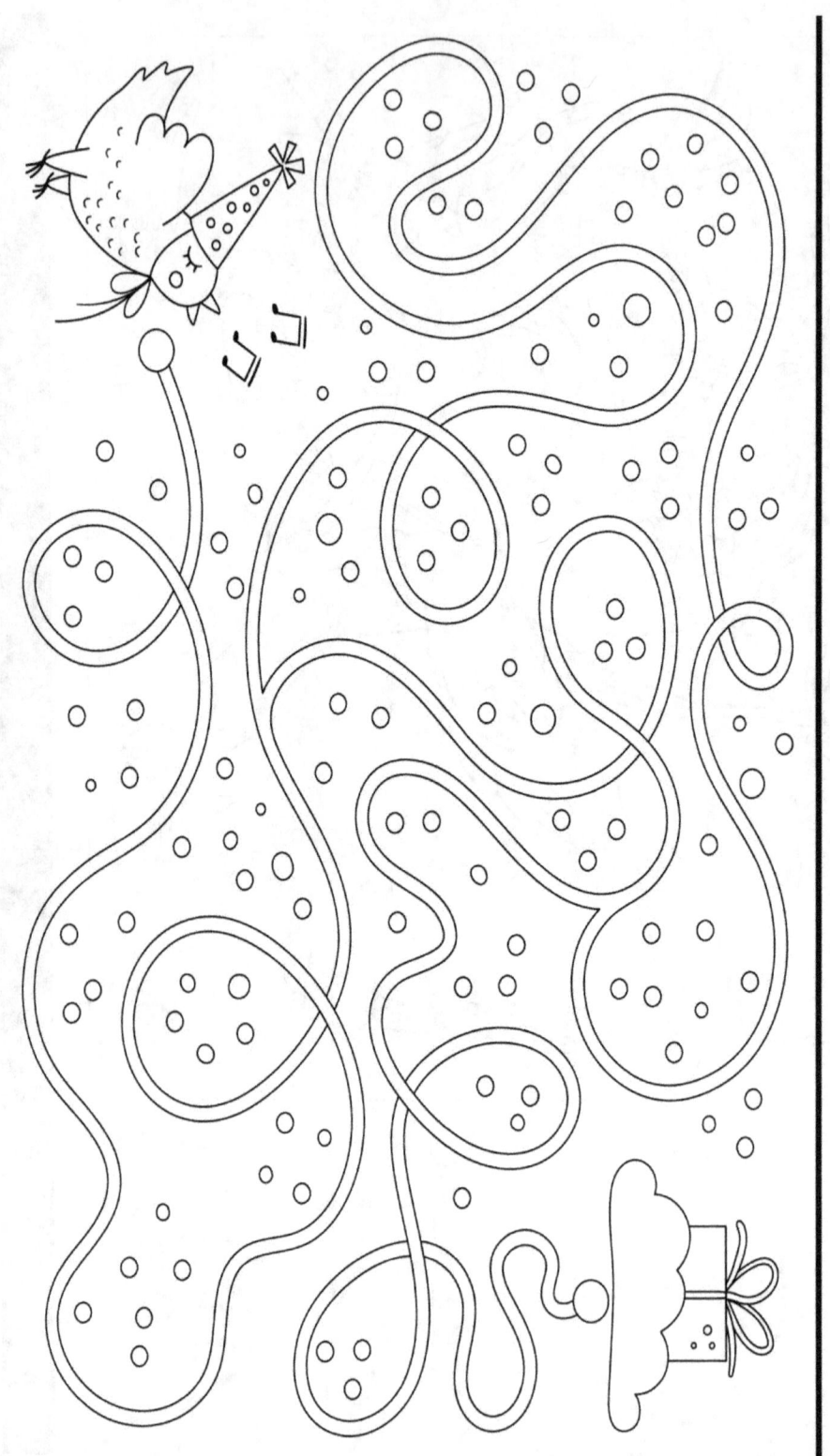

HOW MANY NESTLINGS HAVE HATCHED?

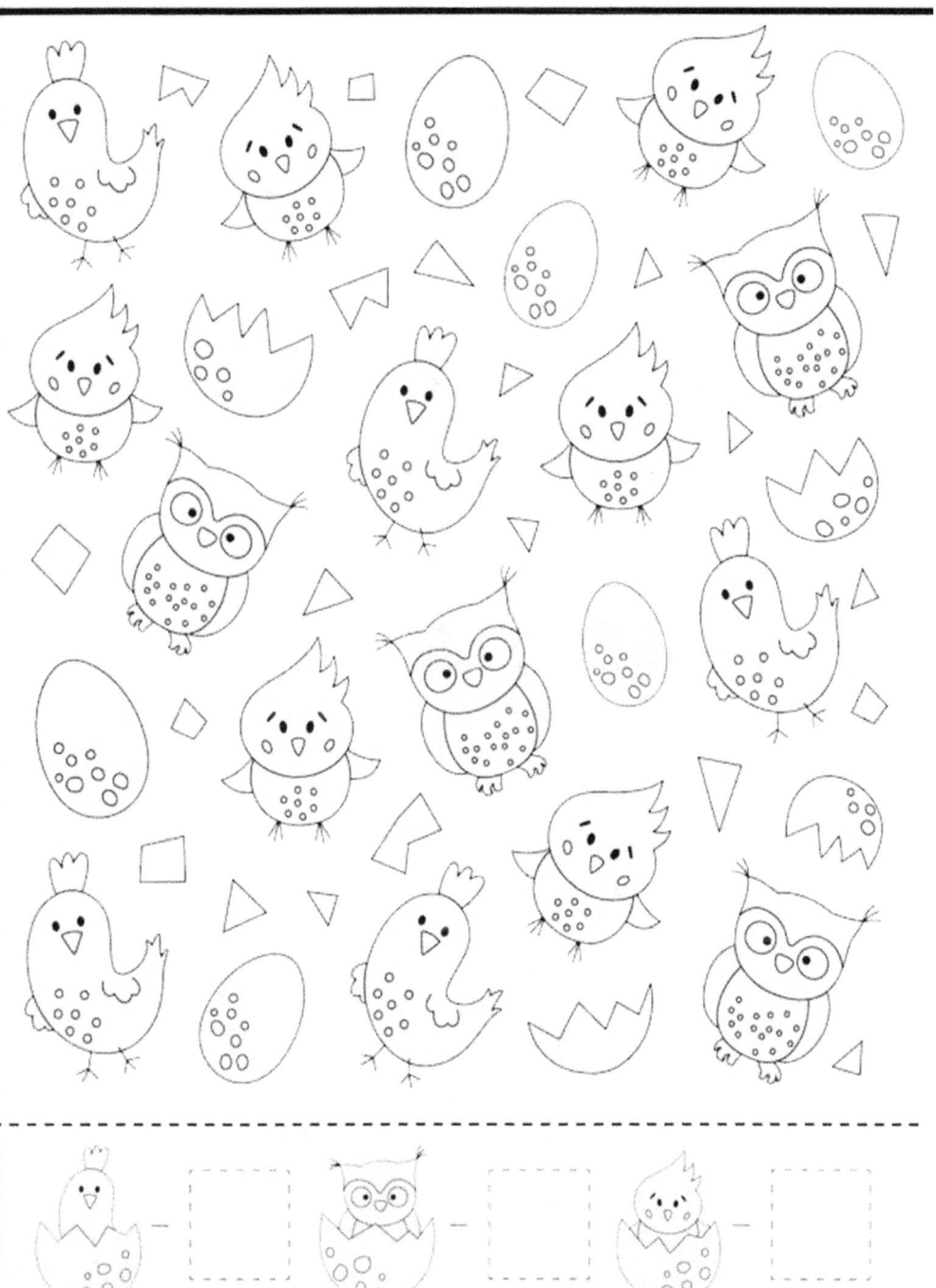

What comes next?

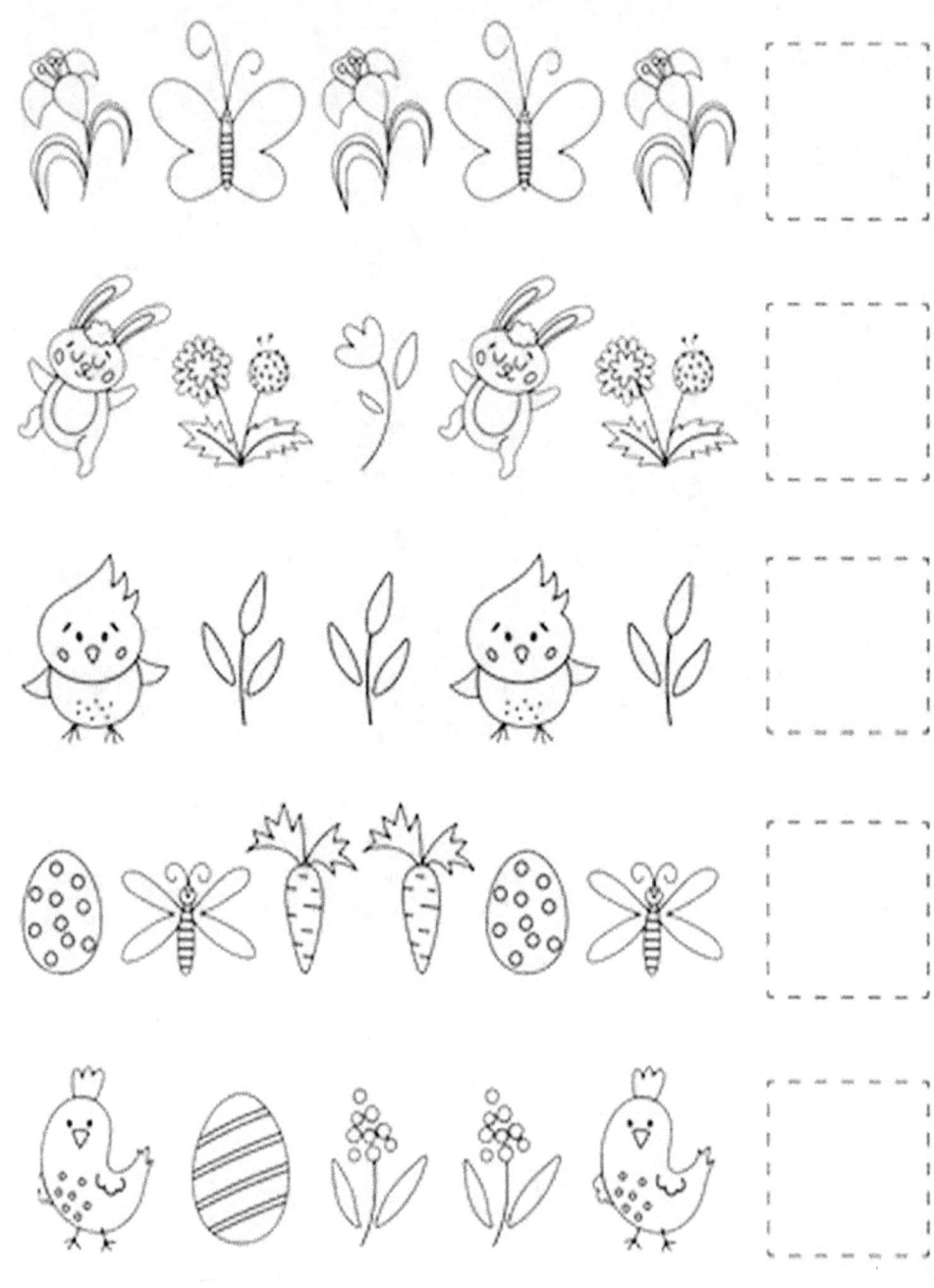

Spot 10 differences

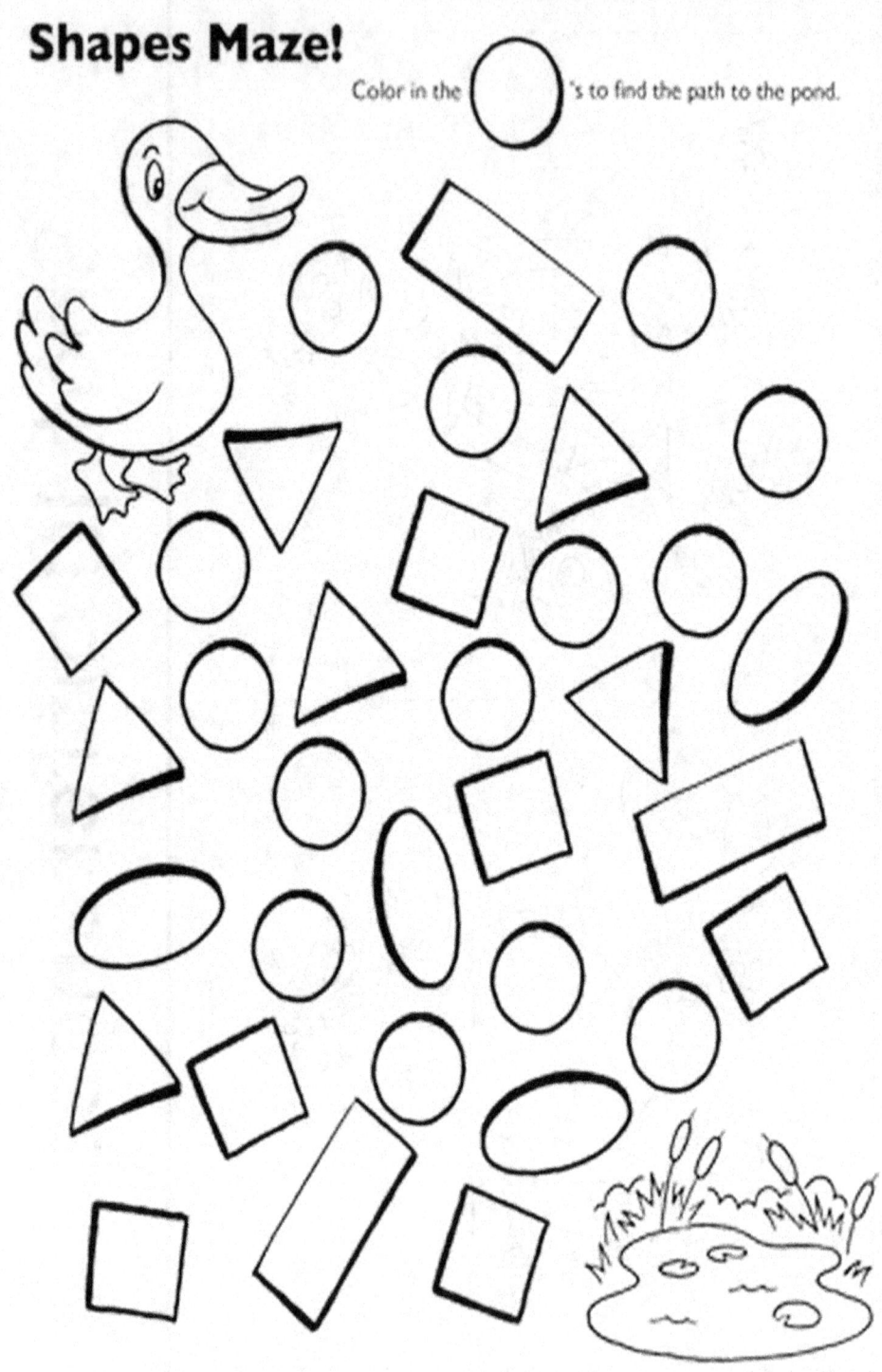

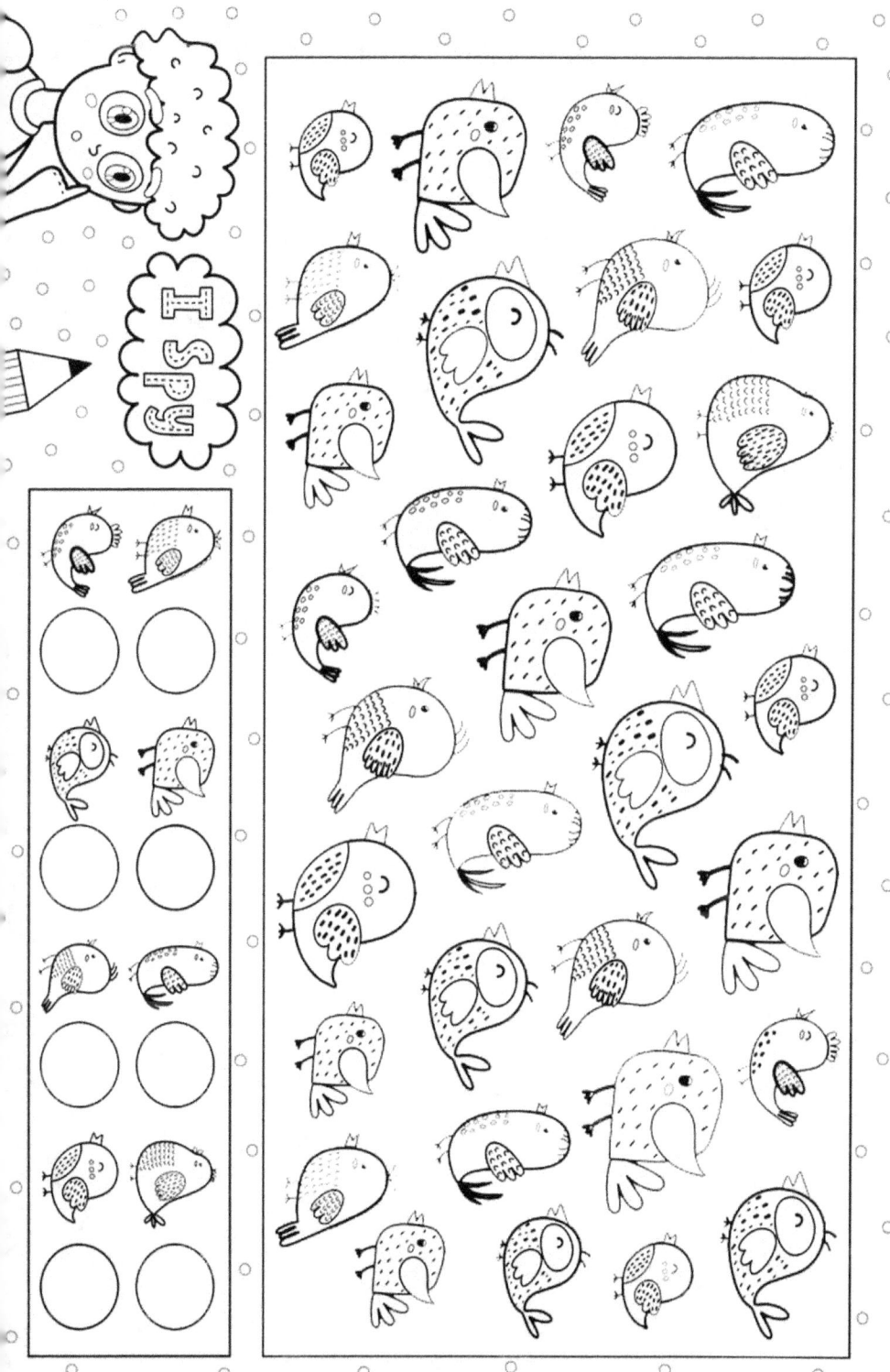

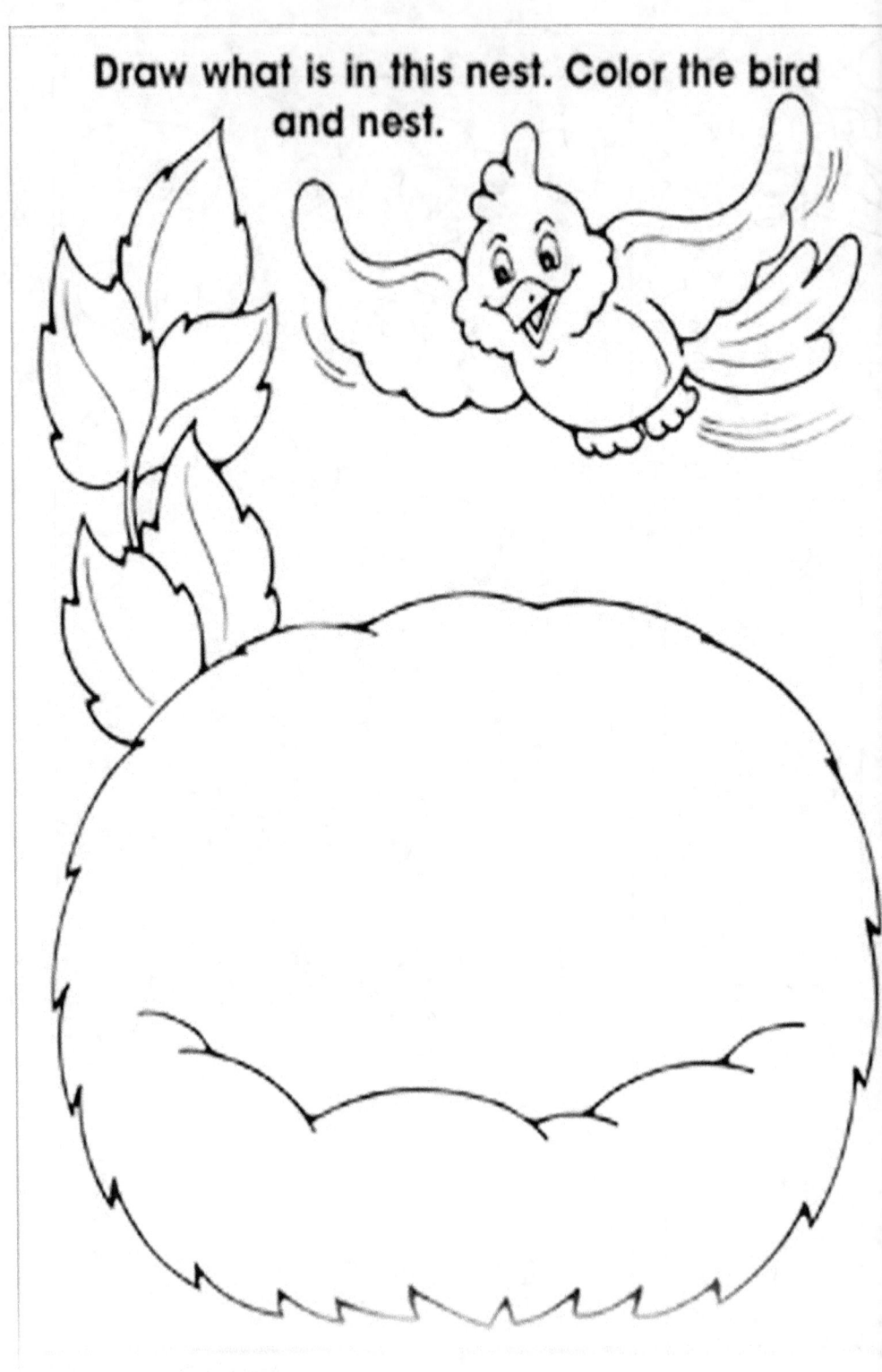

I SPY

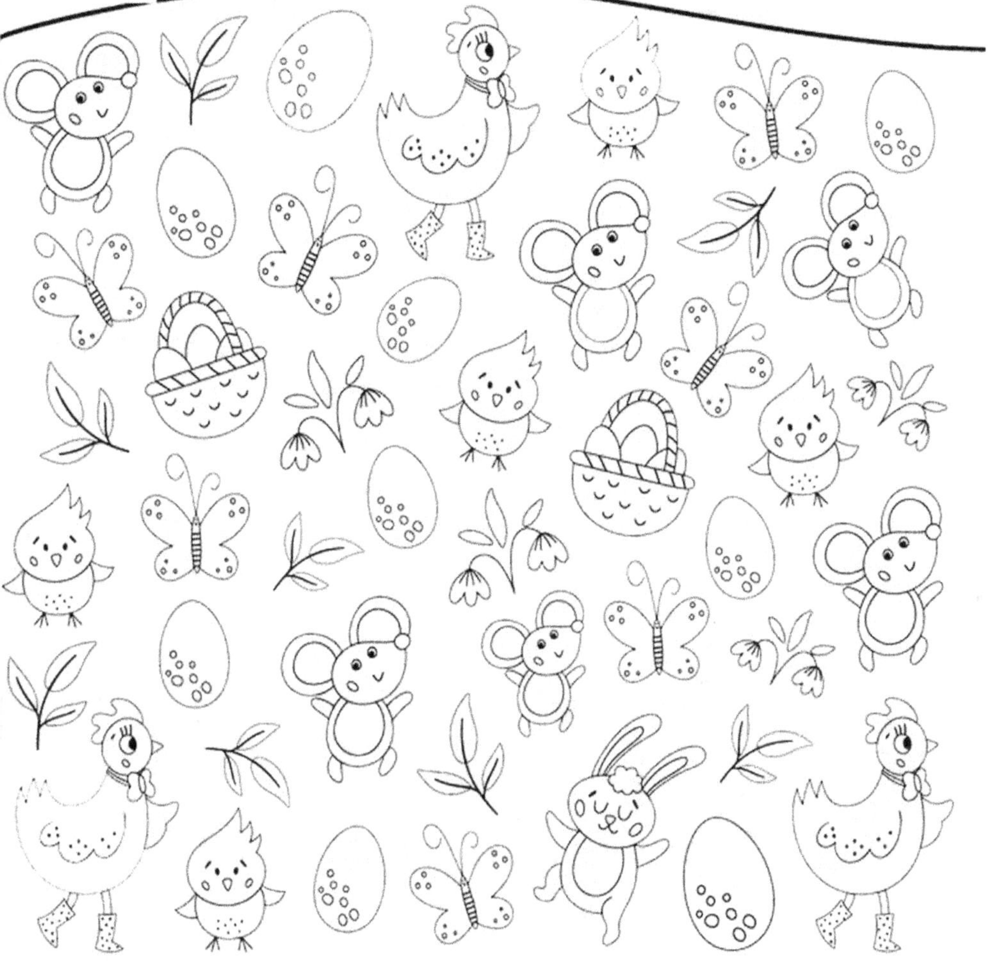

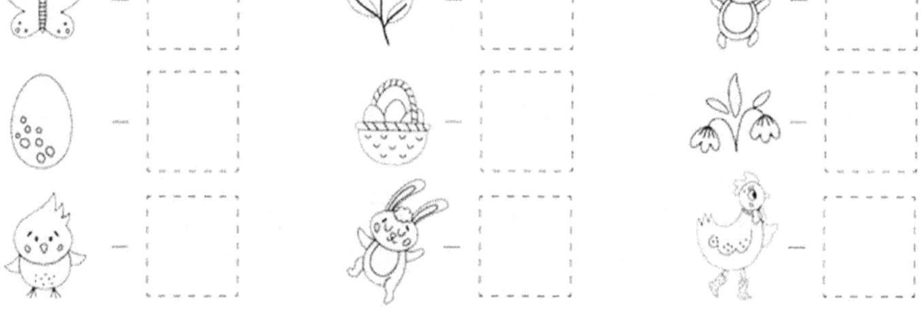

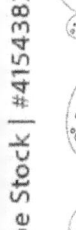
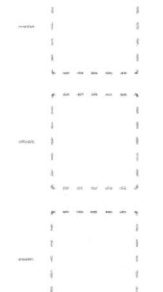
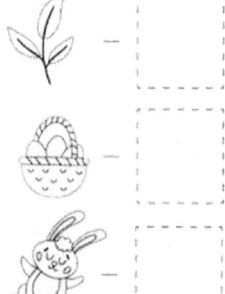
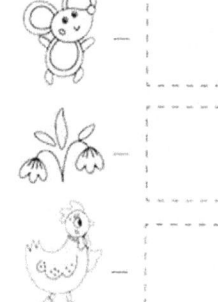

ACTIVITY SHEET

Connect birds with right nests. Count how many eggs are in each nest and write correct number in box below.

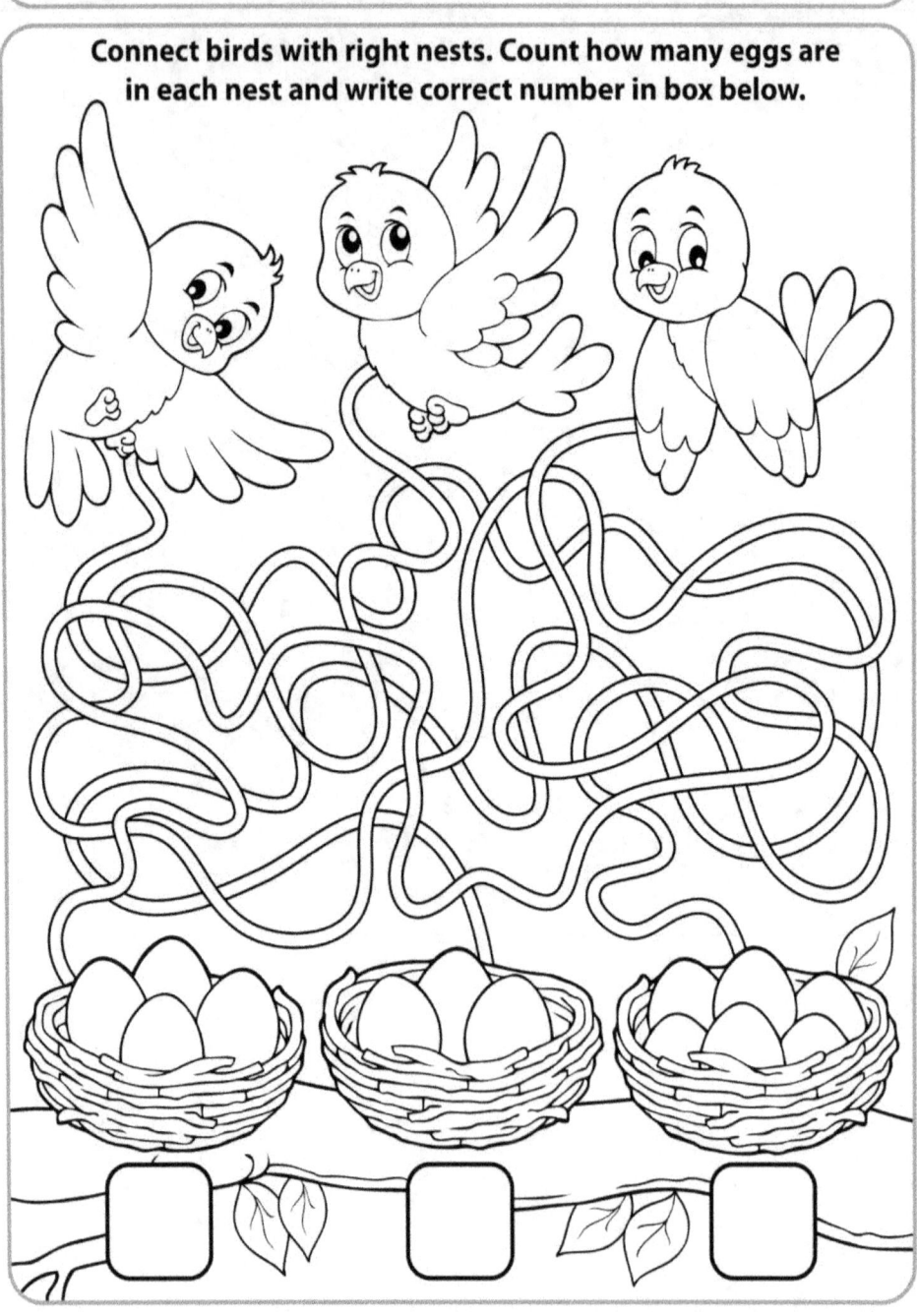

I SPY... Spring

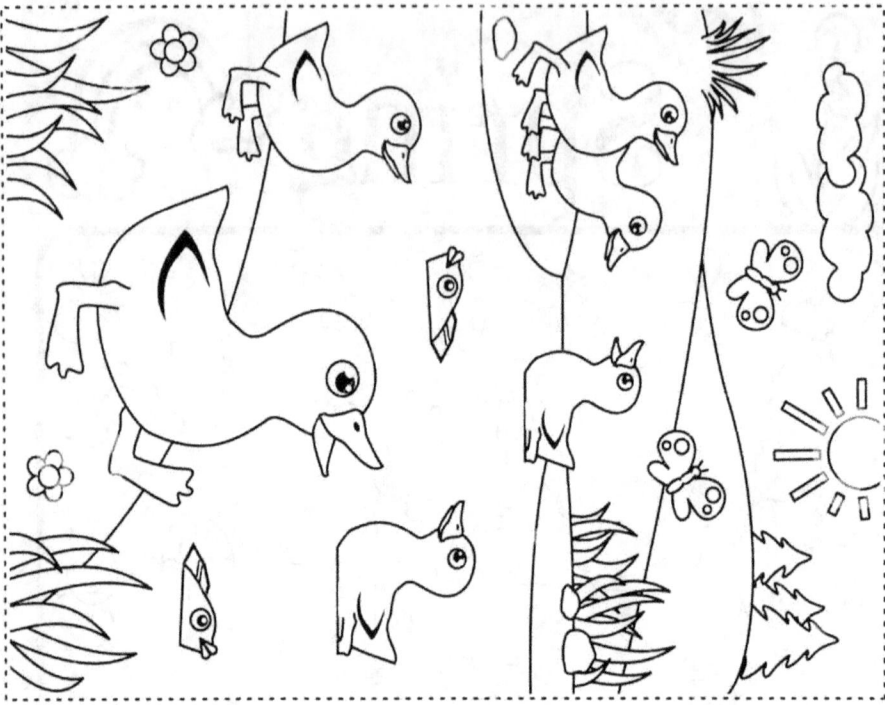

Find the ten differences between the two pictures.

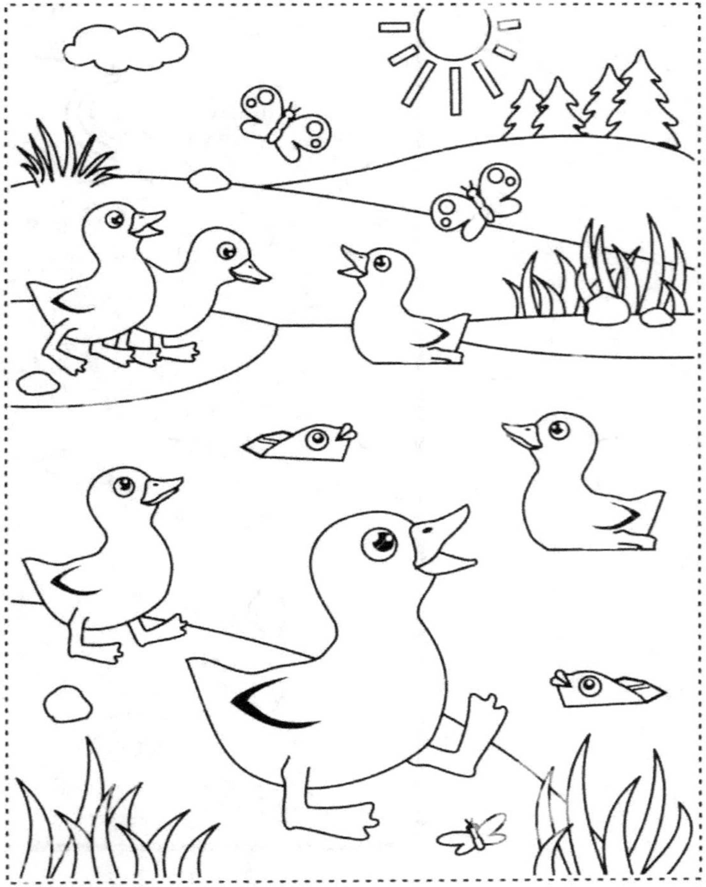

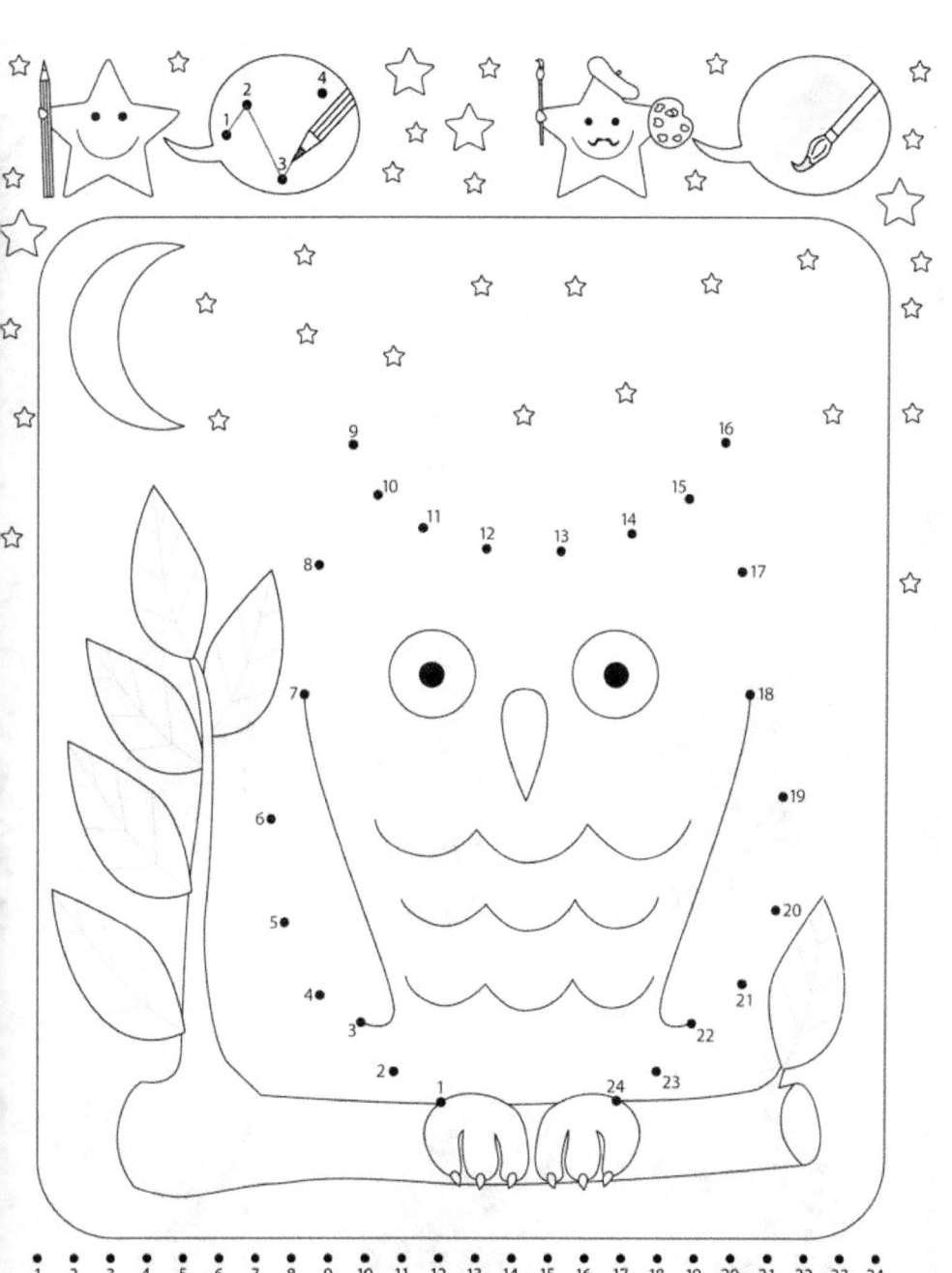

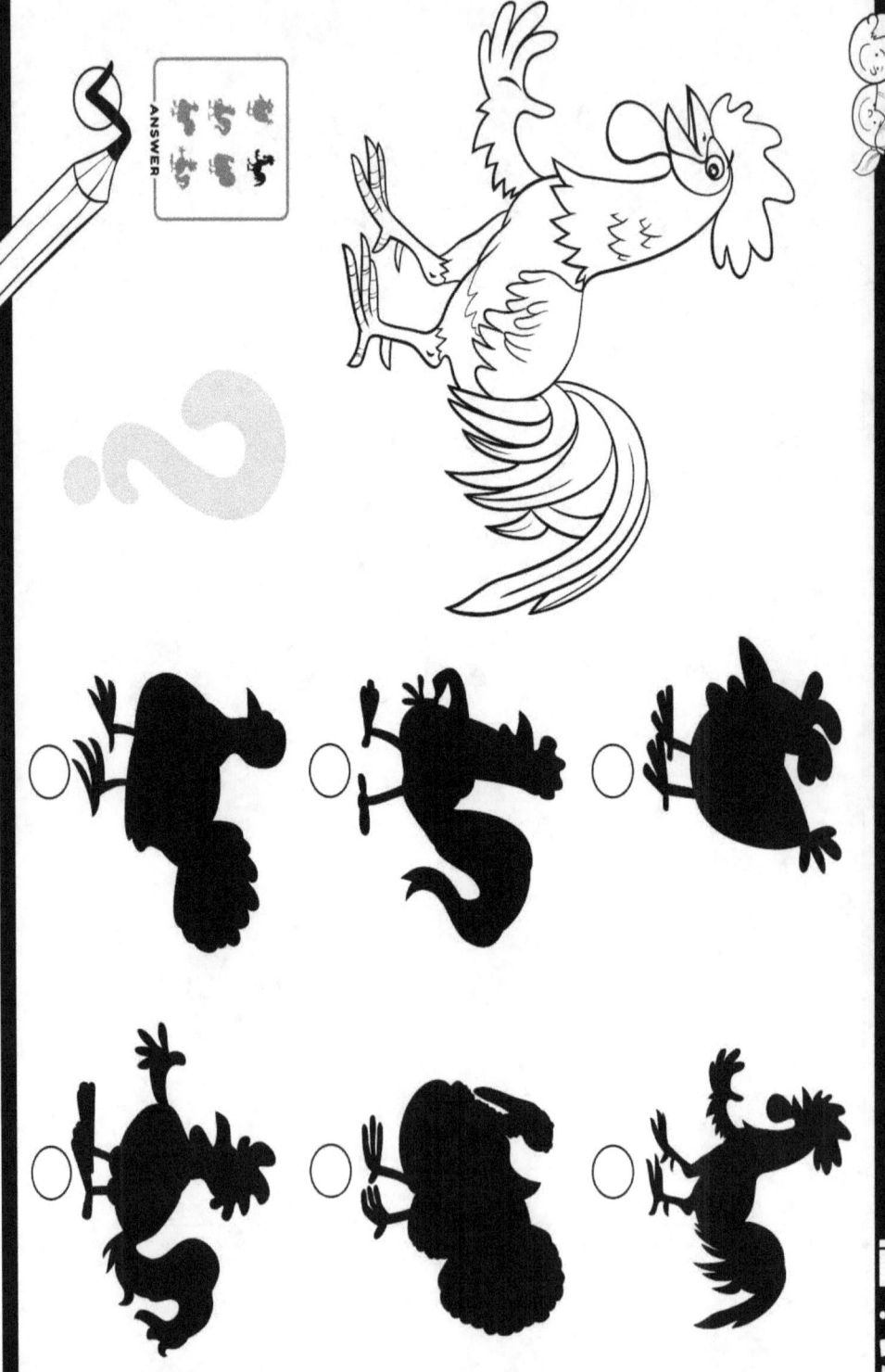

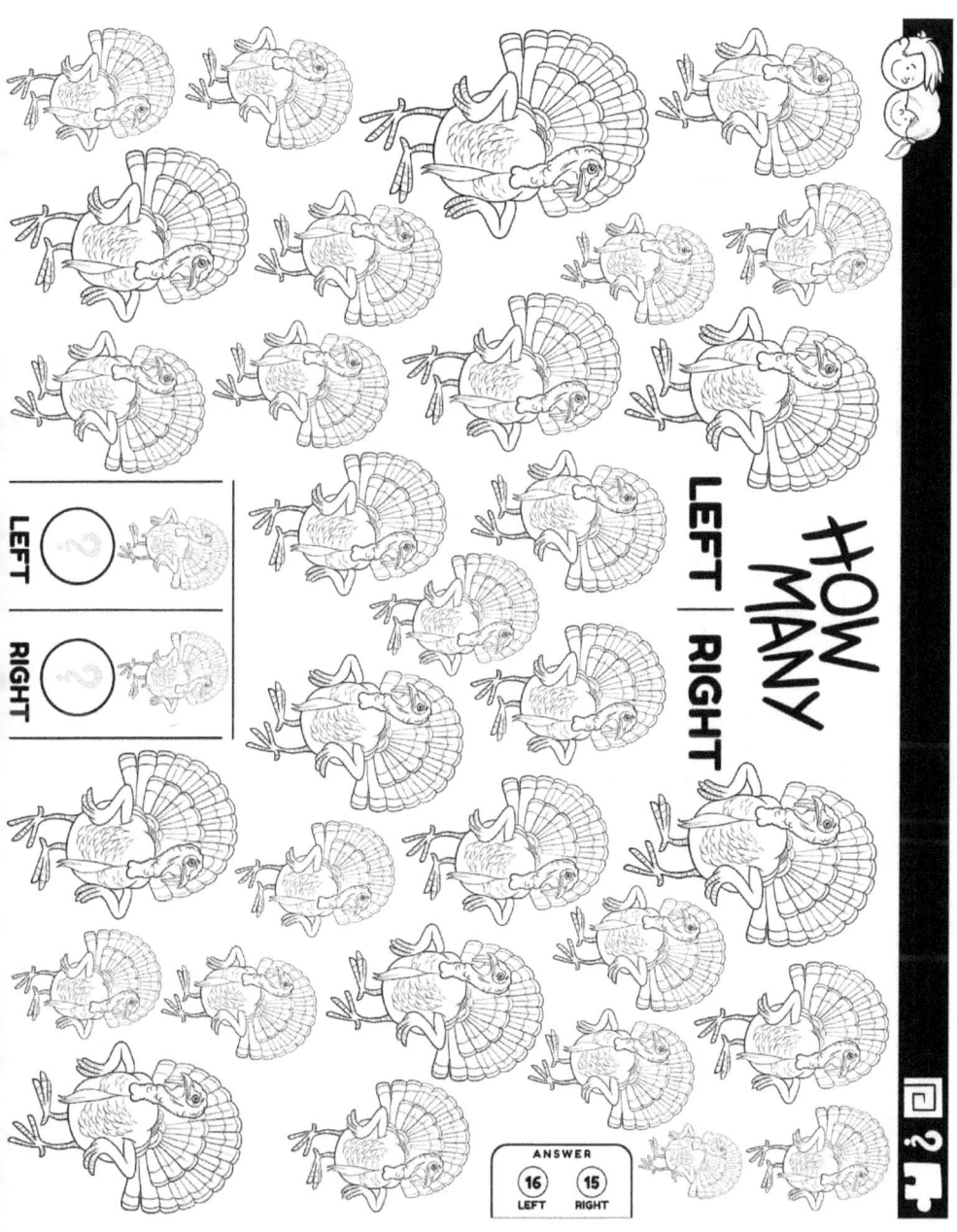

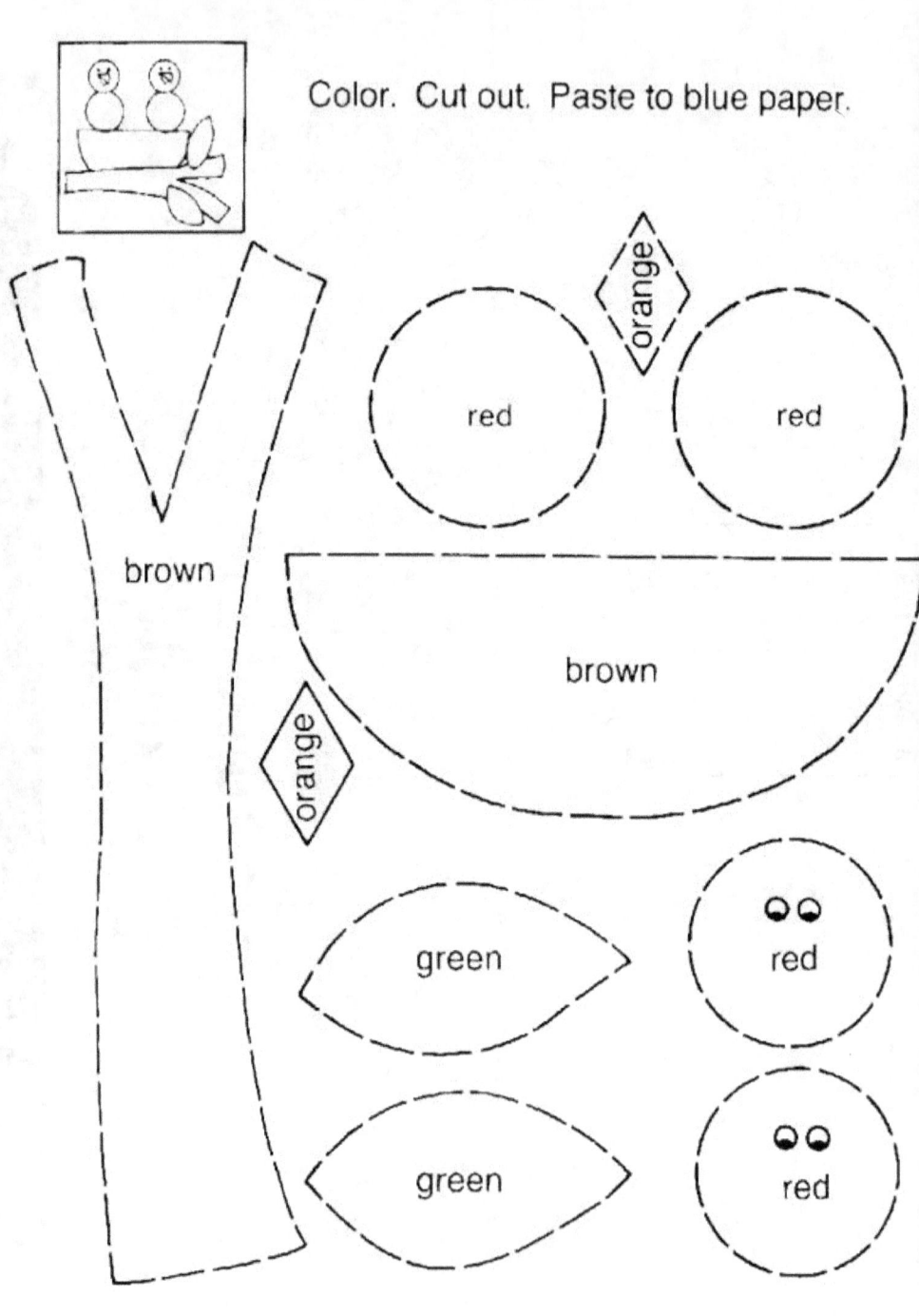

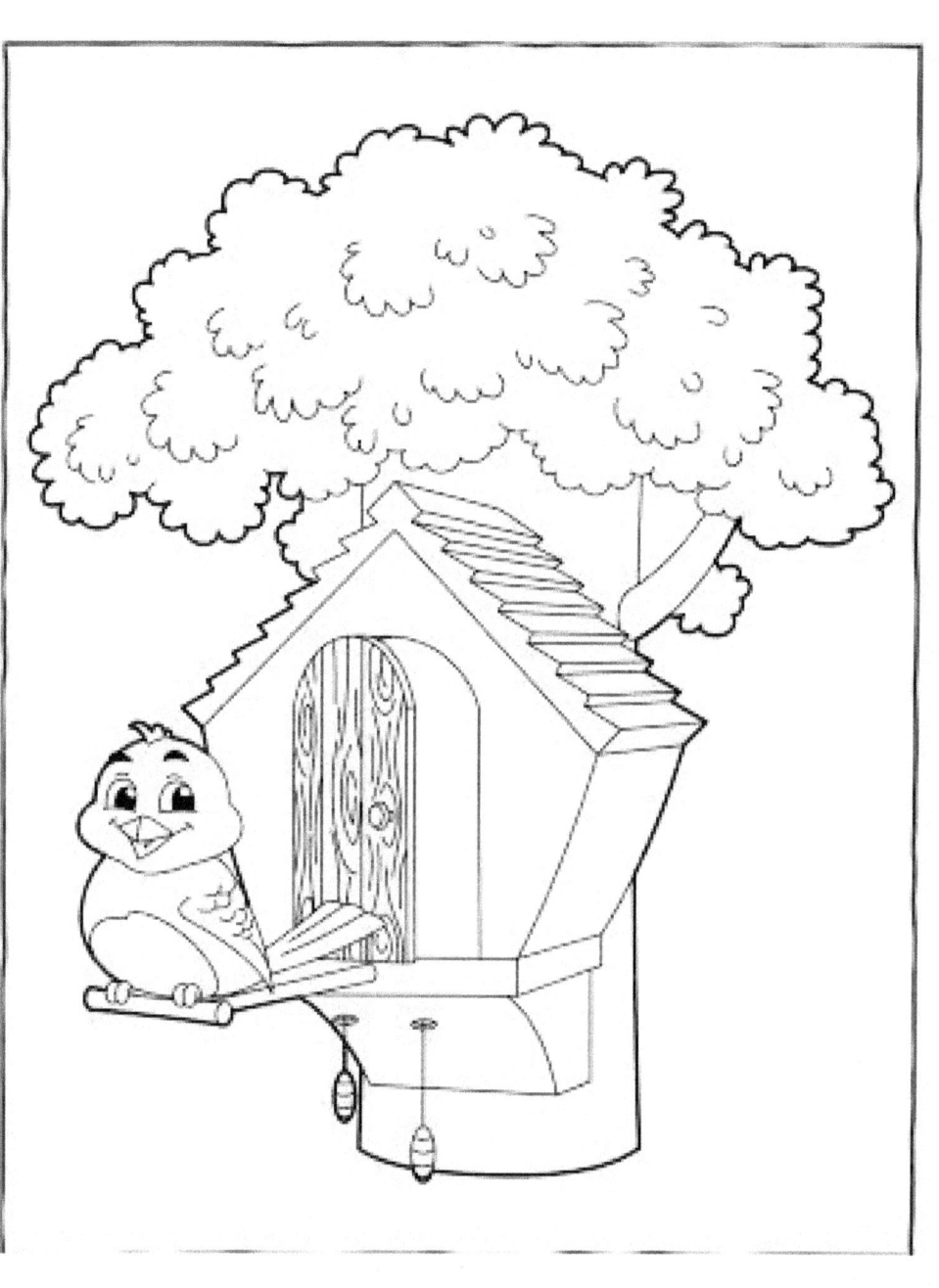

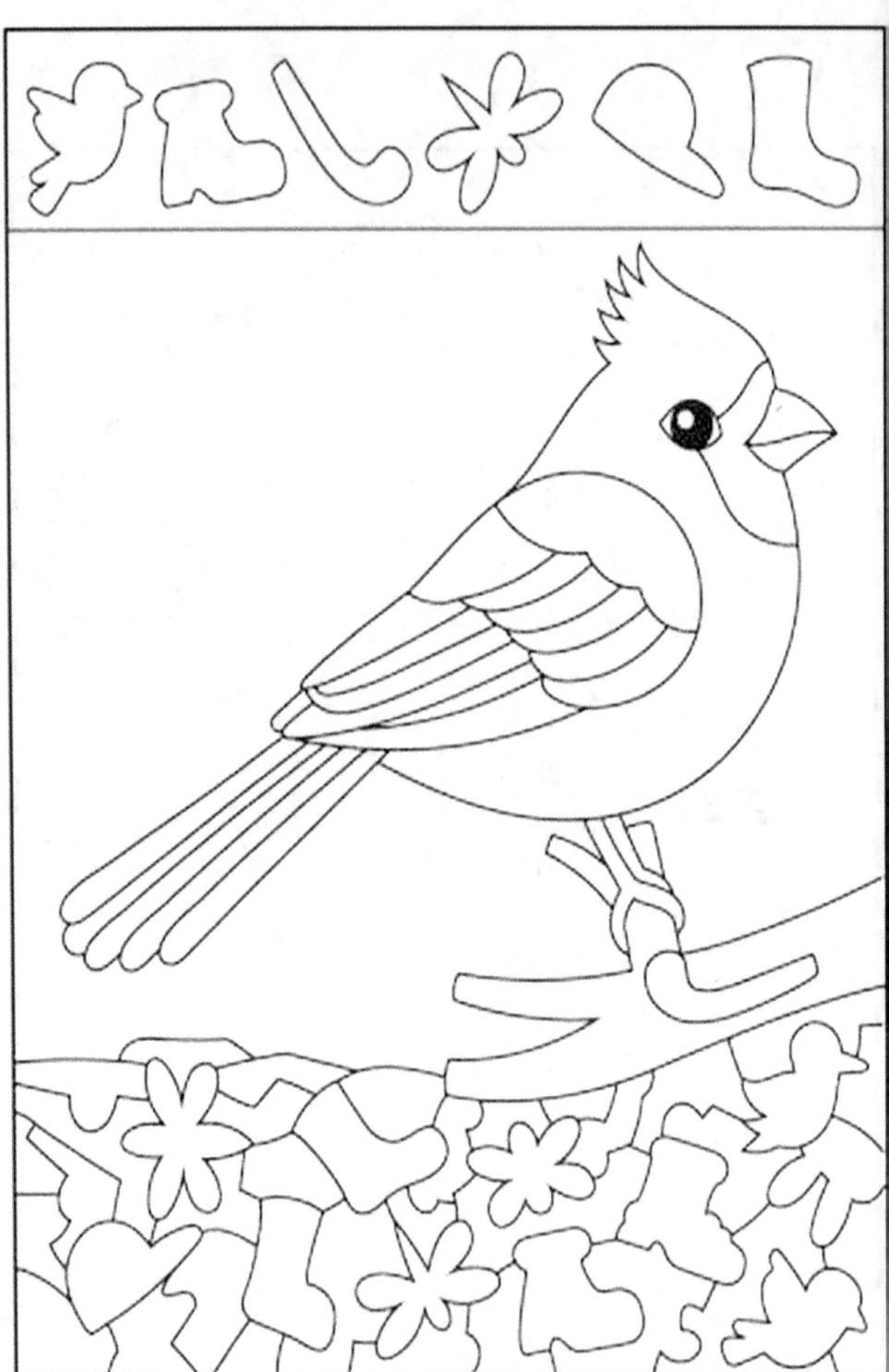

Color the shapes in the owl.

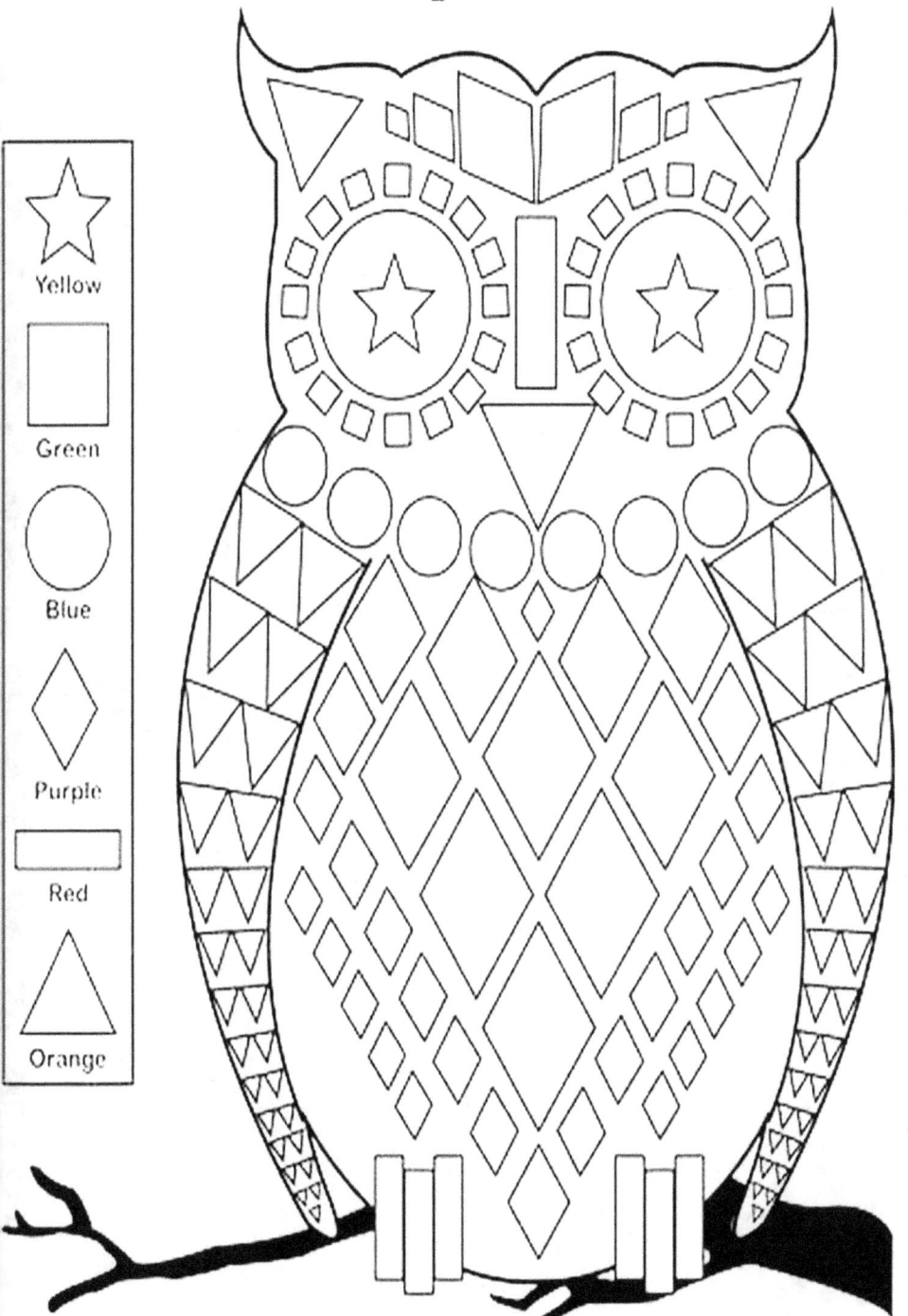

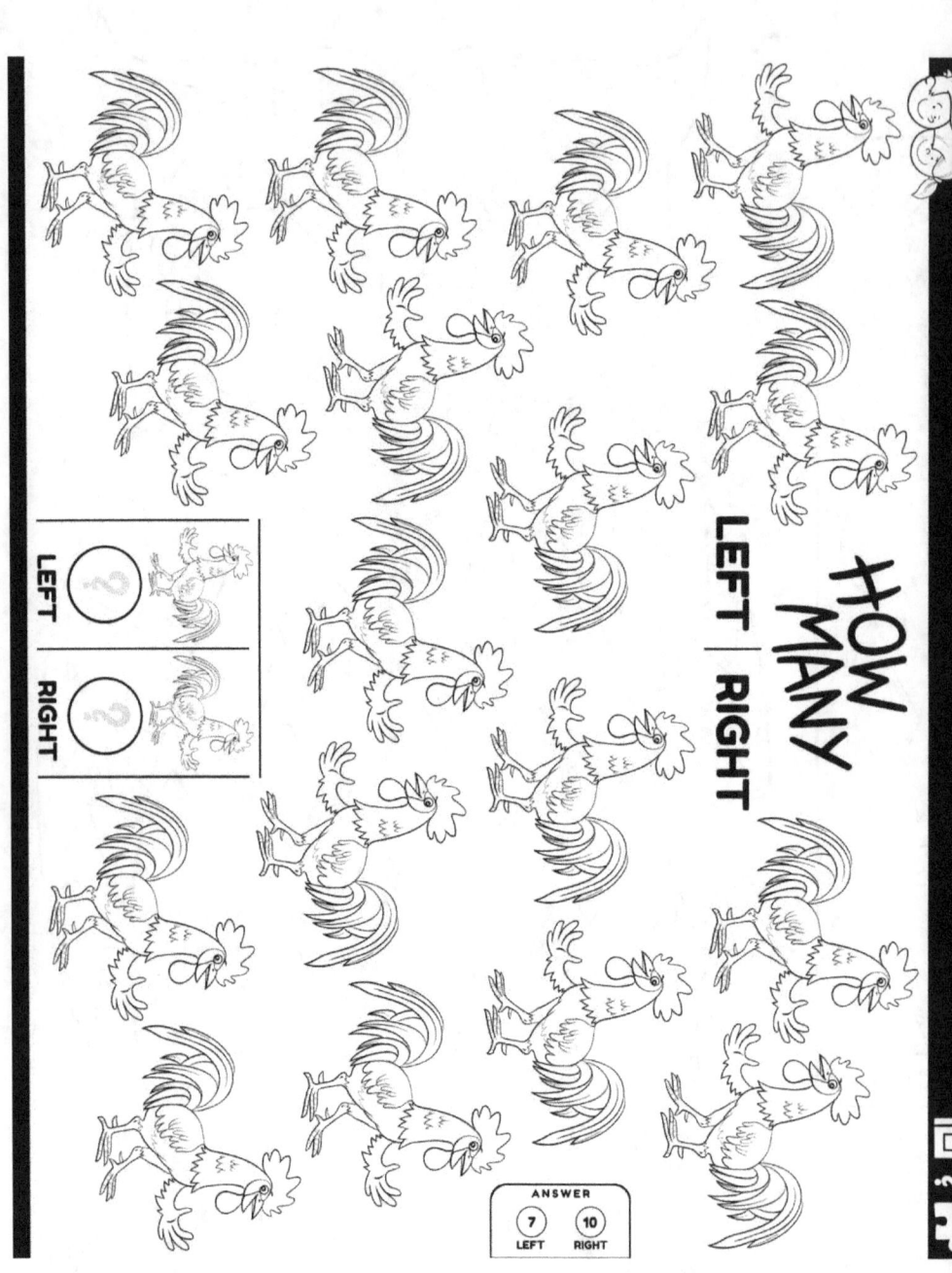

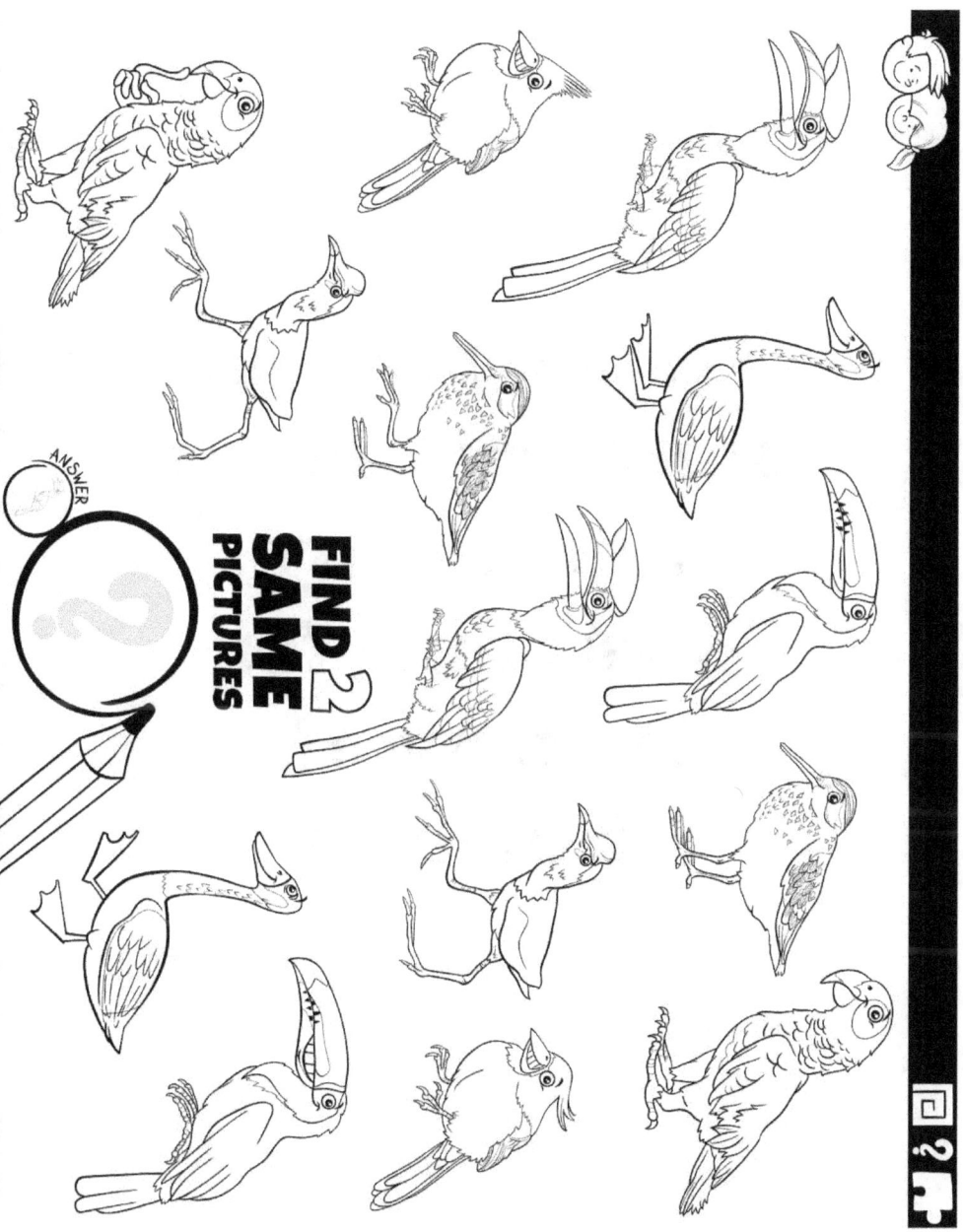

Please see our other listings on Amazon by searching for Homework Helpers!

www.ingramcontent.com/pod-product-compliance
Lightning Source LLC
Chambersburg PA
CBHW070954220526
45471CB00007B/3026